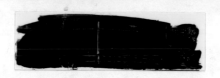

Immunochemical Techniques
Laboratory Manual

Immunochemical Techniques Laboratory Manual

John Goers

Department of Chemistry
California Polytechnic State University
San Luis Obispo, California

Academic Press

Harcourt Brace Jovanovich, Publishers

SAN DIEGO   NEW YORK   BOSTON   LONDON   SYDNEY   TOKYO   TORONTO

This book is printed on acid-free paper. ∞

Academic Press, Inc.

1250 Sixth Avenue, San Diego, California 92101-4311

United Kingdom Edition published by

Academic Press Limited

24–28 Oval Road, London NW1 7DX

Library of Congress Cataloging-in-Publication Data

Goers, John

    Immunochemical techniques laboratory manual / John Goers.

      p. cm.

    Includes index.

    ISBN 0-12-287048-4

    1. Immunochemistry–Laboratory manuals.   2. Immunoassay–

Laboratory manuals.   I. Title.

    [DNLM: 1. Immunoassay–methods.   2. Immunochemistry–laboratory

manuals.   QW 525 G597i]

QR187.I45G64   1993

616.07'56–dc20

DNLM/DLC

for Library of Congress   92-17632

                                                      CIP

PRINTED IN THE UNITED STATES OF AMERICA

92 93 94 95 96 97   EB   9 8 7 6 5 4 3 2 1

Contents

Methods Locator

Preface

This book presents some of the most effective immunochemical techniques used in biology today. The experiments have been thoroughly tested and refined over six years in student laboratories at California Polytechnic State University, and provide dependable protocols not only for students, but also for established research scientists unfamiliar with immunochemical techniques. The experiments are introduced in order of increasing complexity: the first five experiments introduce the "classical" techniques of antibody purification and characterization, while the last five experiments cover more "modern" techniques such as protein blotting, immunoprecipitation, ELISA, immunocytochemistry, and antibody labeling. Thus, the early experiments provide labeled antibody reagents for the later techniques, reflecting a "research" approach that stresses the initial production of specific reagents followed by their application. In addition, the experiments have been carefully designed to require a minimum of expensive equipment and reagents. Except for a microtiter plate reader, the equipment required for the experiments is available in most undergraduate biochemistry laboratories. This will allow even minimally equipped institutions to effectively introduce students to immunochemistry.

The experiments in this book may be incorporated into either a quarter- or a semester-long course with two three-hour laboratory sections per week. The Suggested Schedule provided may be most easily modified after the third week. Many of the experiments are performed simultaneously to accommodate the many redundant incubation steps of an earlier experiment with new material from the next experiment. This integration of several overlapping experimental procedures has worked quite well—as long as adequate pre-lab explanation is given—and provides an exciting laboratory experience, as completed results often stimulate further experimentation.

It is strongly suggested that students have a background in immunology and biochemistry from either previous or concurrent lecture courses. These students will be able to fully appreciate the approach and discussion of the experiments and will be able to effectively incorporate this knowledge into new protocols. I encourage instructors to expose as many students as possible to immunochemistry and to take the initiative to help dedicated, enthusiastic students who may not have the optimal background. Immunochemistry is so critical to modern biotechnology that as many students as possible should know the fundamental techniques presented in this manual. Furthermore, the practical experience gained from this course helps students find employment in the burgeoning biotechnology industry; former students have told me they were able to secure desirable employment because of this course.

I hope this manual provides a basis for immunochemical laboratory courses in schools previously hesitant to offer such courses. I encourage those interested in developing such a course with my conviction that students need this information to effectively contribute to and integrate into the world of biotechnology. I would be happy to share ideas and answer questions related to any part of this text.

Finally, I would like to acknowledge a few people whose ideas and support continue to guide me to this day. Verne Schumaker stimulated me with his clever interpretation of experimental results and clear deductions. Rodney Porter encouraged me to develop new insights into a problem by combining my research with results from different fields. Tom McKearn and John Rodwell supported my attempts with new career experiences and helped me realize my present position. And perhaps I owe my most warmth and gratitude to the one person who sweetens my life daily, Alison.

John W. F. Goers

Notes to Students and Instructors

1. Student Background for Laboratory

The experiments in this manual have been designed for students with a background in biochemistry and immunology. Typically, this includes advanced undergraduates or beginning graduate students who have had a survey course in immunology that covers the cells involved in the immune response, antibody structure, theory of antigen–antibody interactions, and the use of immune reactions in science.

Students who have not studied immunology are at a disadvantage. Because they are unfamiliar with antibody structure and the immune system, these students will have difficulty following both the rationale of these experiments and the use of the various reagents. An instructor may partially compensate for such a deficit by expanding the prelaboratory lectures to include basic immunology principles. However, the experiments take up a considerable portion of the laboratory period, and there may not be enough lecture time to adequately address the background material.

2. Immunochemistry Supplies Needed for this Laboratory Course

The experiments in this manual may be done with equipment available in most biochemistry teaching laboratories. Equipment that may *not* be available in biochemistry laboratories are a microtiter plate reader (for ELISA assays), an electrotransfer cell (for Western blotting), and a light microscope (for viewing stained cells).

Below is a partial listing of supplies necessary to perform the experiments, assuming a class size of 16 students working in groups of two. This list is not meant to be exhaustive, but will help in determining the minimum supplies required for the course. *All* equipment and supplies necessary for the experiments are listed at the beginning of every experimental protocol, and suggested vendors and stock numbers are included for critical items. Additional vendors and their product lines are listed in Appendix E.

Supplies	Experiments
Animals Mice are used as a source of splenic lymphocytes in Experiment 9. The animals may be inbred or in-house hybrids.	9
Balance Analytical (milligram range) Preparation (gram range) Minimum of one per laboratory classroom.	2-III, 4, 5, 6
Centrifuges Clinical (for isolation of spleen leukocytes) Microfuge (for washing of microsamples) Superspeed, refrigerated (for isolation of immunoglobulin)	2, 3, 8, 9
Chromatography column For isolation of IgG by DEAE. A fraction collector is not necessary since the fractionation is complete within 3 hr.	2-I
Coldbox or large refrigerator Storage of many solutions, protein fractions, and dialysis beakers requires a minimum of one refrigerator.	All
Conductivity meter Needed to verify salt concentration following dialysis. *Not* required.	2-I
Electrophoresis apparatuses Polyacrylamide gel electrophoresis (PAGE) and Western blotting require one vertical slab gel (preferably of mini gel size) per student group. Immunoelectrophoresis (IEP) requires one horizontal apparatus per student group, which may be either a commercial IEP apparatus or a horizontal agarose or cellulose acetate apparatus.	2-II, 4-II
Freezer –20°C for laboratory short-term storage; –70°C for long-term storage of antisera and antigens.	All
Fume hood Needed for cyanogen bromide activation of affinity matrix.	5-I

continues

Supplies	Experiments
Ice machine Students should be constantly aware of keeping protein samples cold during experimentation.	All
Microscope A phase contrast scope capable of 1000×. Photographic capabilities not necessary but are useful. A minimum of one per laboratory classroom.	9
Microtiter plate reader Needed for the ELISA for quantitative results. Not absolutely necessary if the goal of the experiment is to present *qualitative* appreciation of the assay. The results are usually obvious by simply noting the color differences between well columns.	10
Power supply unit Used for three procedures: PAGE, IEP, and Western blotting. The unit must be capable of 0–200 V and 0–200 mA. The minumum number of units needed will vary depending on the number of outlets per unit and the number of simultaneous electrophoresis runs.	2-II, 4-II, 7-II
Reciprocating shaker Not essential, but very useful for preparing affinity matrix, washing of blot membranes, and staining of PAGE gels.	2-II, 5-I, 7
Spectrophotometer Single- or dual-beam UV spectrophotometer. Wavelength- and time-scanning capabilities *not* necessary. Minimum of two spectrophotometers per class, but the more the better. Remember to have quartz or "disposable" plastic methacrylate cuvets that are transparent down to 280 nm.	2, 3, 5, 6
Transfer unit Used to electrotransfer proteins from PAGE gel to cellulose nitrate membrane during Western blotting. Many sizes are available, and usually blots from an entire class may be prepared with one apparatus having two 15 × 20-cm holders.	7-II
Waterbath 37°C used for enzyme incubation during IgG fragmentation and for general quick thawing of protein solutions	2-III + general

3. Antibody Requirements for Experiments

Source of Antibody

The sequence of experiments begins with the purification of antibody from serum and ends with experiments that use this antibody in various immunoassay procedures. The entire progression of experiments requires a substantial amount of an antiserum to a specific antigen, about 10–15 ml per pair of students. Thus, it is prudent to consider which antigen will be used throughout the course and the cost of the antiserum. There is no easy way out of this problem: instructors must either purchase the antiserum or produce it.

Nevertheless, commercial sources of small amounts of labeled antibodies are all that is required to expose students to the use of labeled antibodies as probes in the enzyme-linked immunosorbent assay (ELISA), immunoblotting, immunocytochemical staining, and immunoprecipitation procedures presented in Experiments 7–10. The use of relatively large quantities of antiserum can be avoided in this manner, but students will miss learning about purification (Experiments 2 and 5), characterization (Experiments 3 and 4), and labeling of antibodies (Experiment 6).

Choice of Antigen

Glucose oxidase (mw 80,000) and transferrin (mw 70,000) are the two antigens that have been used successfully in the experiments in this manual. Other possible antigens include: bovine immunoglobulin G (mw 150,000), yeast glucose-6-phosphate dehydrogenase (mw 55,000/subunit), *E. Coli* ß-galactosidase (mw 135,000/sub-unit), and calf intestine alkaline phosphatase (mw 80,000). The last three antigens have the advantage of being enzymes, the activity of which may be inhibited by specific antisera. These antigens were chosen for the following reasons, which should be primary considerations in an introductory immunochemistry course.

1. The antigen should be inexpensive, commercially available, and in a form pure enough for immediate immunization. The minimum amount of antigen necessary for a successful immunization of one goat ranges from 5

Notes to Students and Instructors

to 20 mg. Costs of the antigen must also include the use of the antigen throughout the course in the various asssay procedures.

2. The antigen must produce a high titer antiserum. I would suggest using protein antigens, since they consistently induce a strong immune response.

3. The antigen should have properties that are suitable for the laboratory experiments. The molecular weights should be suitable for PAGE separation, and the stability of the antigen should include resistance to denaturation upon freeze/thawing, stability at room temperatures, and compatibility with Tris or phosphate buffers. If possible, the antigen should have an enzymic or binding function that may be easily monitored. Experiments exploring the effects of antibody binding on antigen function are then possible.

4. The antigen should be nonpathogenic and of bacterial or animal origin. Avoid human antigens, since the source of the antigen for subsequent assays require both the use of human tissue or serum and considerably more attention to safe handling practices.

5. The antigen cannot originate from the same species as the immunizing animal. If an antigen is known to be a poor immunogen, increasing the phylogenetic distance between the antigen and immunizing animal will result in a stronger immune response.

Commercial Sources of Antibody

There are a number of immunology companies that provide custom polyclonal antisera production. The antisera produced will have high specificity and titer as long as sufficient pure antigen that is known to elicit a good response is used. The cost ranges between $1000–3000 to provide 1 liter of antisera. If each student pair receives 10 ml, the cost of antiserum per pair is moderate, ranging from $5–$15 per student. The advantages of custom antisera are substantial; little effort is required of the instructor except to provide the antigen, which may be purchased in pure form. However, the instructor must plan far enough in advance to allow the

6–9 months production time before the laboratory course begins. Companies that provide custom polyclonal antiserum production are listed in Appendix E.

Animals for Production of Antisera In House

The production of antiserum at a university is not a difficult task, but it is time-consuming and redundant. Furthermore, depending on the facilities of the university, the cost of housing, feeding, and caring for an animal over six months to a year may be considerable. Be sure to determine these costs before embarking on your own immunization program.

The best animals for immunization are sheep and goats. Both animals are hardy, provide large amounts of serum, and respond well to a wide variety of antigens. If the institution cannot support a sheep or goat, then the rabbit is the next best animal of choice. However, several rabbits and significantly more effort in obtaining blood is required to obtain the same amount of antiserum resulting from one sheep or goat. Detailed information on the preparation of antigen for immunization and the immunization process is given in Appendix H.

4. Suggested Schedule of Experiments

Experiment	Week 1	Week 2	Week 3	Week 4	Week 5
1	day 1				
2-IA	day 1 / day 2				
2-IB		day 1 / day 2	day 3		
2-II			day 1 / day 2		
2-III		day 1 / day 2			
3		day 1	day 2		
4-I		day 1	day 2		
4-II			day 1 / day 2		
4-III			day 1	day 2	
5-I				day 1 / day 2	
5-II					day 1

Experiment	Week 6	Week 7	Week 8	Week 9	Week 10
6-I	day 1 / day 2				
6-II	day 1				
7-I		day 1 / day 2			
7-II			day 1 / day 2	day 3	
8		day 1 / day 2	day 3 / day 4		
9				day 1 / day 2	
10			day 1 / day 2	day 3 / day 4	day 4

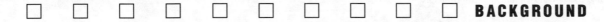

Review of the Immune System and Immunoglobulin Structure

This section briefly will review the immune system from two perspectives: cellular interactions and antibody structure.

Some Definitions

Antigens and Epitopes

An *antigen* is a substance capable of being recognized and bound by the immune system. Antigens may be whole organisms (bacteria) or individual molecules. Not every part of an antigen interacts with immune system molecules. The parts of antigens that directly interact with antigen receptor molecules (such as antibodies) are called *epitopes*. Most antigens have several epitopes. A *hapten* is a small organic molecule that is able to bind antigen receptor sites, although it is too small to induce an immune response by itself. Nevertheless, it may elicit a strong response if covalently bound to a *carrier*, a high molecular weight immunogenic protein or synthetic polymer.

MHC Complex

The body has a system of marker glycoproteins encoded by a group of genes known as the *major histocompatibility complex* (MHC). These molecules are embedded in the cell membranes of virtually every cell. They are extremely polymorphic, and all individuals, except identical twins and members of essentially genetically identical inbred strains, have unique combinations of MHC proteins.

These proteins are involved in the communication between cells during immune responses and are responsible for the susceptibility of certain individuals to diseases that involve inability to respond to certain types of antigens. Different *classes* of MHC molecules, I, II, and III, exist. Each class is involved in different aspects of immune regulation and is encoded by an extensive gene system.

Cellular Basis of the Immune Response

Immune Cells

Immune cells originate from the leukocyte lineage, and include both lymphoid and myeloid cells (Figure 1). Stem cells originating in the bone marrow migrate to various tissues and mature into different immune competent cells.

T Cells and B Cells

Lymphocytes are small white blood cells primarily responsible for mounting an effective response to an antigen. The two major types are the *B cells* and the

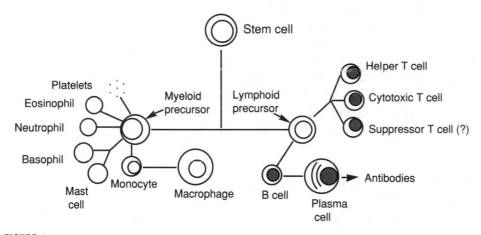

FIGURE 1

Cells of the immune system.

T cells; B cells depend on the bone marrow for their maturation, whereas T cells depend on the thymus. When stimulated by an antigen, B cells respond by secreting soluble *antibodies,* proteins capable of binding to a specific antigen. This is known as *humoral immunity*. T cells respond either by stimulating other immune-associated cells or by directly attacking the antigen, which is usually a foreign cell, a virus, or a cancerous cell. This response is known as *cellular immunity*.

Different types, or subsets, of B and T lymphocytes have distinguishing molecules on their surfaces that are useful for identification, since there are no visible differences between the cells under a microscope. For instance, whereas all T cells carry the CD3 marker protein on their surface, only helper T cells also have the CD4 marker protein, and only suppressor or cytotoxic T cells have an additional CD8 marker protein. A useful B cell marker is surface IgM, which is absent on T cells.

The B and T cells recognize antigens using surface *antigen receptors*. On B cells, the antigen receptor is a membrane-bound antibody molecule (IgM or IgD class). When the B cells bind an antigen, they mature into antibody-producing *plasma* cells. The plasma cells secrete antibody with specificity for the antigen identical to that of the original receptor on the B cell surface. The antigen receptor on T cells is an immunoglobulinlike molecule that must interact with MHC molecules to bind antigen effectively. T cells do not synthesize antibodies when activated; instead, they produce *lymphokines*, low molecular weight substances that act as messengers to signal immune system cells into responses such as target-cell death, macrophage activation, lymphocyte cell growth, and cell migration.

Polyclonal and Monoclonal Response

Each T or B lymphocyte is capable of recognizing only one specific epitope. Thus, in an immune response to a antigen with many epitopes (such as a bacterium with many different epitope molecules on its surface), many different lymphocytes will be activated, each by its specific epitope. Each activated lymphocyte may grow into a clone of identical cells in response to the antigen, resulting in a proliferation of many clones with different specificities, a *polyclonal* response.

For example, as a result of the polyclonal expansion of different B cells in response to one antigen, a number of different antibodies will be produced, each capable of recognizing one particular epitope on the antigen. This results in a heterogenous antibody population directed at the antigen. Scientists have learned to manipulate the immune system to select a *hybridoma,* a cell derived from a single clone of activated B cells that produces a homogeneous *monoclonal* antibody; a single molecular species of antibody to an antigen.

Antigen-Presenting Cells

Antigen-presenting cells (APCs), present antigens to lymphocytes for an effective immune response. Most antigens, although cancer cells and some viruses are examples of exceptions, must be engulfed (phagocytized) by the APCs, broken down by intracellular processes, and finally "presented" on the cell surface in a form that is recognized by lymphocytes. For instance, protein antigens are cleaved into peptides for presentation. The exact nature and reason for this is not clear, but many cells are capable of this process, including (foremost) macrophages, dendritic cells, and even B cells. Macrophages are found throughout the body, especially in the lymphoid tissues (a monocyte is a circulating blood precursor of the macrophage), whereas dendritic cells are in the epidermis and lymphoid tissue.

Immune Response

The immune response to an antigen depends on the type of antigen and the particular cells involved. For simplicity, we will consider the activation of B cells independent of the activation of T cells.

B cells are activated after interaction with both processed antigen and helper T cells (Figure 2). The B cell binds and processes the antigen, presenting it to a helper T cell (CD4+) after the antigen is bound to a MHC class II protein on the B cell surface. (Other APCs may substitute for the B cell during this process.) The T cell then binds the processed antigen and releases appropriate lymphokines, which stimulate the B cell to become an antibody-producing plasma cell. (Interleukin 4 is primarily responsible for B cell growth.) The antibody then binds to the antigen and triggers the activation of *complement*, a series of proteins capable of both directly lysing target cells and attracting phagocytic cells, mostly macrophages, to

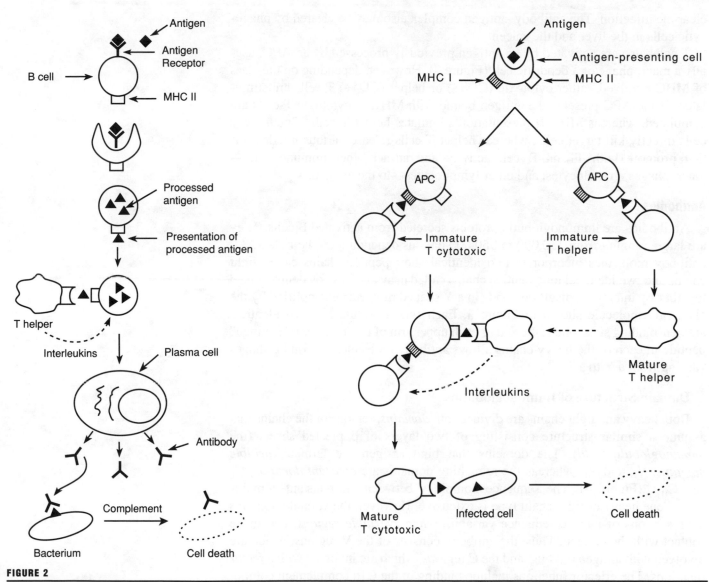

FIGURE 2

(*Left*) B cell activation. (*Right*) T cell activation.

clear the infection. The antibody–antigen complex also may be cleared by phago-cytic cells in the liver and the spleen.

T cells also are activated by an antigen previously processed by an APC, usu-ally a macrophage or a dendritic cell (Figure 2). However, depending on the class of MHC involved, either cytotoxic (CD8+) or helper (CD4+) T cells are stimu-lated. If the APC presents the antigen bound with MHC 1, cytotoxic T cells are stimulated, whereas MHC II presentation stimulates helper T cells. Cytotoxic T cells directly kill target cells, whereas helper T cells release various interleukins that promote both T and B cell activity and attract other immune cells—macrophages, granulocytes, and other lymphocytes—to the antigen.

Antibodies

Antibodies are immunoglobulin proteins secreted from activated B cells. They are large, ranging from 150,000 to 950,000 daltons depending on their class. All antibody molecules incorporate two identical short peptide chains called light chains and two identical long peptide chains called heavy chains covalently linked together by interchain disulfide bonds in a Y-shaped molecule exemplified by the class IgG molecule shown in Figure 3. Each IgG molecule has two identical antigen-binding sites, one at the end of each upper arm of the Y. A flexible "hinge" peptide in each of the heavy chains allows antibody molecules to assume shapes varying from a Y to a T.

Domain Structure of Immunoglobulins

Both heavy and light chains are divided into *domains*, regions of the chains that assume a similar structure consisting of two layers of β pleated sheets (the *immunoglobulin fold*). The domains that bind antigen are termed *variable domains*, V_H and V_L, whereas the remaining domains are *constant domains,* C_L and $C_{H_{1-4}}$ (Figure 3). The sequence homology between the constant domains within one heavy or light chain type is extensive. However, the variable domains have sections of intense sequence variability, *hypervariable regions,* that make contact with the antigen. Thus, the antibody consists of the V regions, which are involved with antigen binding, and the C regions, which are involved with *effector* functions. The effector functions include binding of the C1q complement compo-

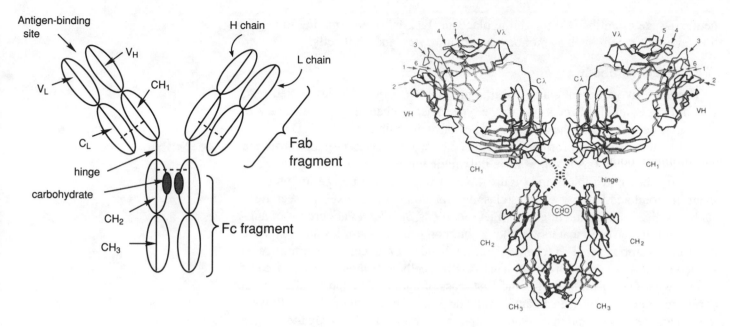

FIGURE 3

Heavy and light chain structure of IgG class antibody. (*Left*) The heavy and light chains are divided into domains, areas of the polypeptides that have a similar structure consisting of two layers of β sheets. These domains are designated V (variable) or C (constant). The V domains bind the antigen, whereas the C domains are responsible for *effector* functions such as binding to specific cell receptors and activation of complement. The dashed lines represent interchain H–L disulfide bonds. Intradomain disulfides are present in each domain, but not shown. (*Right*) This view of IgG shows more detail of the polypeptide structure and a more realistic orientation of the H and L λ chain domains. The antigen binding sites are composed of "loops" of both V_H and V_L (numbered 1–6), which make direct contact with the antigen. These are hypervariable in sequence and give rise to the designation *variable* domain. Reprinted with permission from *Nature*, **349**, 294. Copyright ©1991 by Macmillan Magazines Limited.

nent, passage of antibody through the placenta (IgG only), and binding to receptors on effector cells such as monocytes, granulocytes, and mast cells.

Classes of Antibody

There are five different classes of immunoglobulin molecules designated IgA, IgG, IgD, IgE, and IgM according to the type of heavy chain they possess, α, γ, δ, ε, or μ. All classes share the same two types of light chains, κ and λ. IgD and IgE have the same overall conformation as IgG (Figure 3) with one Y-shaped structure per molecule, while IgA and IgM have polymeric forms of the Y-shaped structure, which are shown in Table 1 and Figure 4. Classes IgG, IgM, and IgA are predominant in blood and tissues, whereas class IgA predominates in external secretions such as saliva, mucus, and intestinal tract secretions. *Subclasses* are groups of antibodies within one class that have either a common structure—for instance, all have the same number of H–H chain disulfide bonds—or a common amino acid sequence. IgM occurs both on the surface of B cells as a *monomer* and free in serum, where as a *pentamer* it is the first class of antibody to appear after initial exposure of an individual to an antigen. Its large number of binding sites allows it to bind antigen avidly and to activate complement efficiently to destroy the antigen quickly. IgG is the most concentrated immunoglobulin in serum; it is the predominant class of antibody produced on repeated exposures to an antigen. IgA occurs in highest concentration in secretions such as those of the mucosal lining of the gut. IgA is transported across the endothelium only after attachment of two additional peptide chains to two IgA "monomers": the *J chain* and the *secretory component*. The J chain binds two monomers of IgA into a dimer; the secretory component promotes transport of the dimer across the cell membrane. The function of IgD is not known precisely, but it does occur on the surface of B cells and may be involved with regulation of antibody production. IgE occurs in very low concentration in serum, but is known to occur on the surface of *mast cells,* cells involved in the swelling characteristic of allergic reactions.

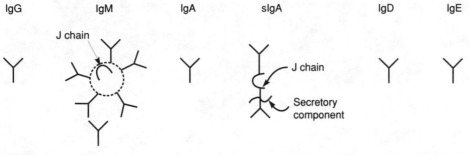

IgG   IgM   IgA   sIgA   IgD   IgE

J chain

J chain

Secretory
component

FIGURE 4

Schematic structures of classes of antibodies.

TABLE 1

Properties of Human Immunoglobulins

Class	H chain	Number of domains in H chain	L chain	Molecular weight ($\times 10^3$)	Antigen-binding sites per molecule	Average serum concentration (mg/ml)	Subclass designations
IgG	γ	4	κ,λ	150	2	20	IgG1,2,3,4
IgM	μ	5	κ,λ	950	2 or 10	1–2	none
IgA	α	4	κ,λ	160 + (dimer)	2 or 4	0.5	IgA1,2 and sIgA
IgD	δ	4	κ,λ	170	2	0.05	none
IgE	ε	5	κ,λ	190	2	0.0002	? or none

Preparation of Serum from Blood

Immunization involves injecting an animal with an antigen to elicit an immune response. Normally, immunization results in the production of specific antibody molecules capable of recognizing and binding the antigen. These molecules accumulate in the blood of the animal and are used as reagents for immunological techniques, many of which are presented in this laboratory manual. This experiment presents the first step to isolate the antibody molecules from blood, the separation of serum from blood.

When the blood is collected and allowed to sit, the clotting proteins convert soluble fibrinogen into cross-linked fibrin, which entraps blood cells and forms a gel-like mass called a clot. If the clot is allowed to sit for a time, it contracts, forcing the cells and the fibrin into a denser mass and squeezing other soluble proteins into a fluid known as *serum*. Serum contains all the soluble blood proteins, except the active clotting factors and fibrinogen, and is often the starting material from which blood proteins, including antibodies, are purified.

When serum is electrophoresed, its proteins separate into a number of broad components termed the α, β, and γ globulin regions, as well as the predominant albumin peak (Figure 1-1). Albumin constitutes more than half of total serum protein and migrates far toward the positive pole (anode) because of its high negative charge. It is an acidic protein with an isoelectric point, pI, of 5, reflecting the large number of carboxyl-containing amino acid side chains. Conversely, γ globulins are basic proteins because they have a large number of amino-containing amino acids, causing their pIs to be near 8.0. They have a net positive charge at neutral pH and migrate slightly toward the negative pole (cathode). The separation of serum into these five major regions masks the huge number of different proteins in serum: at least twenty major ones with hundreds of others in minute concentrations (Table 1-1).

In our experiments, we will be studying and using the serum proteins known as *immunoglobulins*. These proteins commonly are called *antibodies* and migrate in the γ globulin region.

Albumin is very soluble in water, whereas a globulin is insoluble in pure water. Globulins are most soluble in 0.05–0.2 M solutions of neutral salts, such as NaCl or Na_2HPO_4, but may be "salted out" with 2–3 M solutions of other neutral salts such as ammonium sulfate or sodium sulfate.

TABLE 1-1

Major Human Serum Proteins

Protein	Molecular weight (kDal)	Average concentration (mg/ml)	Electrophoretic mobility	pI	Function
Prealbumin	54	0.25		4.7	thyroxine binding
Albumin	66	44			maintaining osmolarity; ion, lipid, and drug transport
α_1-Lipoprotein	200	2.5	α_1		lipid transport
α_1-Antitrypsin	55	2.9	α_1	4.0	protease inhibitor
Ceruloplasmin	100	0.3	α_2	4.4	Cu binding; oxidase
Haptoglobin	100	1.6	α_2	4.5	hemoglobin binding
α_2-Macroglobulin	800	2.5	α_2	5.4	protease inhibitor
β-Lipoprotein	~3000	1.0	β_1		lipid transport
Hemopexin	57	1.0	β_1		heme binding
Transferrin	77	2.9	β_1	5.8	iron transport
Complement C4	206	0.25	β_1		complement component
Complement C3 (β_1c-globulin)	213	1.1	β_2		complement component
Fibrinogen	340	3.0	β_2	5.8	precursor of fibrin clot
IgA	160	2.1	γ		antibody
IgM	1000	1.5	γ	5.1–7.8	antibody
IgG	150	12.5	γ	5.8–8.3	antibody

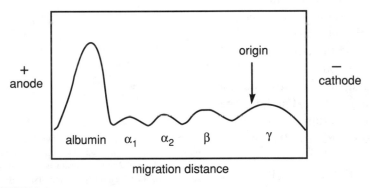

FIGURE 1.1

Electrophoresis of serum at pH 7. Adapted from Tietz (1986).

Experiment

In this exercise, the preparation of nonimmunized control serum from blood is described. The serum will be used in later experiments as a source of immunoglobulin for nonspecific antibody controls.

Materials

□ freshly drawn nonimmunized sheep or goat blood, immediately adjusted to 0.01 M EDTA, pH 7.4, to prevent clotting (also available commercially in Alsevers preservative solution from Colorado Serum, Rockland, and Pelfreeze)

□ 15-ml glass or plastic centrifuge tubes, capable of withstanding 2000 g

□ refrigerated centrifuge

□ thromboplastin (optional)

Procedure

DAY ONE

1. Place freshly drawn blood in centrifuge tubes. Allow to clot 20–30 min. at room temperature or overnight at 4°C.

2. Separate the clot from the serum by either of two methods, centrifugation or filtration.

   a. Centrifuge at 2000 g (about 5000 rpm in an SS34 or JA-21 rotor) for 10 min. Pour off the supernatant (serum) carefully. If loose blood cells are recovered, repeat centrifugation. Freeze at –20°C; add sodium azide to 0.02% if stored at 4°C for more than 1 day.

   b. Filter the serum from the clot by pouring the clotted blood into a funnel with a wad of glass wool at the bottom. The glass wool retains the clot and allows the serum to drip into a tube. The clot slowly retracts during the filtration, releasing more serum, so filtration is most efficient if carried out overnight in a refrigerator. Any cells remaining in the serum

The serum obtained has an active complement system, a system of proenzymes that may be activated by antibody–antigen complexes. The activated complement system releases a number of active products, including opsonins, chemotactic factors, and lytic complexes that may interfere with *in vitro* cell-based assays. Denature several complement components to reduce such interference by heating serum for 10 min. at 59°C.

Blood that clots with difficulty may clot more quickly in glass tubes. If EDTA or citrated blood is being used, add $CaCl_2$ to 50 mM to reverse the effect of the anticoagulants, which chelate Ca^{2+} and inhibit conversion of prothrombin to thrombin.

Thromboplastin may be added to decrease clotting time for sera that clot with difficulty. It helps to run a wooden stick around the inside of the tube to dislodge the clot and allow the clot to shrink for 10–15 min. If you are in a hurry, this step may be omitted.

Speed and time are not critical, unless you are very concerned with hemolysis or cell contamination in the serum. Hemolysis occurs if the blood is allowed to clot for too long a time, or if it is stirred vigorously. If all leukocytes must be removed, recentrifuge the serum for 20 min. at 10,000 rpm.

This type of serum preparation is especially useful for large volumes of blood, when centrifugation is kept to a minimum.

must be pelleted by centrifugation. Freeze serum at $-20°C$; add sodium azide to 0.02% if stored at $4°C$ for more than 1 day.

REFERENCE

Tietz, N. L. (1986). "Textbook of Clinical Chemistry." Saunders, Philadelphia.

Purification and Analysis of IgG

In Section I of this experiment, the immunoglobulin G (IgG) fraction of anti-glucose oxidase will be isolated from serum by salt precipitation and ion exchange chromatography. In Section II, IgG will be analyzed for purity and subunit structure by polyacrylamide gel electrophoresis. Section III continues the analysis of IgG structure using the production of antibody fragments with proteases. The experiment also incorporates precipitation methods from Experiment 4 to assess the presence and purity of IgG. The techniques are discussed separately; each discussion gives an overview of the technique followed by an experimental section.

I. Purification of IgG

A. AMMONIUM SULFATE PRECIPITATION

When serum is electrophoresed, it separates into several broad peaks containing a wide variety of protein (see Figure 1.1). The broad γ globulin region contains a number of different antibody classes: IgA, IgD, IgG, IgE, and IgM. The classes differ in molecular weight, but all have similar protein structure and are capable of binding antigen. Because of their similarity in structure, all classes of antibody precipitate as nondenatured salt complexes between 40 and 50% wt/vol. saturated ammonium sulfate (40–50% SAS). Smaller amounts of albumin, α globulins, and β globulins also precipitate, but the vast majority of precipitated protein is γ globulin. The high concentration of ammonium sulfate causes protein precipitation by competing for solvent water molecules. Water molecules bind to proteins through hydrogen bonds, keeping proteins in solution. If the ammonium sulfate attracts enough water away from the proteins, the proteins lose their water of solvation and come out of solution. Normally, this occurs without gross structural changes in the protein and is a gentle method of removing protein from solution

The concentration of ammonium sulfate is given either in terms of % saturation or in molarity. Usually, it is more convenient to use % saturation, especially when diluting saturated ammonium sulfate to achieve the desired concentration.

Polyethylene glycol also may be used to precipitate a wide variety of proteins, including immunoglobulins (Ingham, 1990).

(England and Seifter, 1990). Protein precipitates often are stored for months to years at 4°C; most often, however, they are dissolved in buffer and dialyzed or gel filtered to remove residual ammonium sulfate. Because ammonium sulfate saturation has little dependence on temperature (3.90 M at 0°C and 4.04 M at 20°C), it is not necessary to control temperature carefully during precipitation. Sodium sulfate at 13–15% saturation also has been used to precipitate γ globulins. However, since the saturation of sodium sulfate varies considerably between 0 and 20°C, it is crucial to control temperature closely when using this salt.

Two methods generally are used to achieve the high concentration of ammonium sulfate required for protein precipitation. In the first method, solid ammonium sulfate is added slowly to a stirred protein solution. Stirring is necessary to avoid localized high concentrations of ammonium sulfate that may cause precipitation of nonimmunoglobulins. In the second method, an amount of SAS is added to the stirred protein solution to achieve the desired saturation percentage. This method avoids the weighing of solid ammonium sulfate, but results in larger volumes of final protein solution for centrifugation. For this reason, when precipitating large volumes of protein, solid ammonium sulfate is used to maintain low centrifugation volumes.

Experiment

First, the γ globulin fraction of anti-glucose oxidase serum will be isolated by ammonium sulfate precipitation. This fraction then will serve as the starting material for the isolation of IgG by DEAE ion-exchange chromatography.

Materials

□ anti-glucose oxidase serum, produced in sheep, goat, or rabbit

□ saturated ammonium sulfate

□ Bring about 800 gm ammonium sulfate up to 1 liter with water; stir at room temperature until mostly dissolved, about 1 hr. Adjust final volume to 1 liter. Adjust the pH to 7 with HCl or NaOH. Filter through #1 filter paper into a reagent bottle. Store at 4°C.

□ 0.05 M potassium phosphate buffer, pH 8.0

Antibodies in polyclonal antiserum will precipitate over a range of 35–50% SAS because of the different molecular species of antibodies present. However, monoclonal antibodies usually precipitate completely after reaching a precise percentage of SAS because if their homogeneity of structure.

Grams of Ammonium Sulfate Added to 1000 ml Protein Solution to Achieve Varying Percentages of Saturation at 0°C.[a]

$(NH_4)SO_4$		$(NH_4)SO_4$	
%	gm	%	gm
20	106	60	361
25	134	65	398
30	164	70	436
35	194	75	476
40	226	80	516
45	258	85	559
50	291	90	603
55	326	100	797
55	326	100	797

Source: Dawson, *et al.* (1986).
[a]Complete table in Appendix F.

☐ super speed centrifuge, capable of 10,000 rpm

☐ 50-ml centrifuge tubes

☐ UV spectrophotometer

☐ conductivity meter

Procedure

DAY ONE

1. Obtain 10–15 ml antiserum from the instructor. Freeze 0.2–0.5 ml serum for analysis in Experiments 2-II and 4-I, II and for protein determination. For this crude protein determination, assume 1 mg/ml protein to have an absorbance of 1.0 at 280 nm.

   > Because serum consists of may different proteins, the extinction coefficient of 1 (mg/ml)$^{-1}$cm^{-1} offers only a rough estimate of protein concentration. An accurate protein determination may be obtained by using a chemical protein assay such as the Lowry, Bradford, or bincinchoninic acid (review and procedures in Stoscheck, 1990). Premixed reagents are available from many biochemical suppliers including Bio-Rad, Sigma, and Pierce (see Appendix E).

2. Add an equal volume of SAS to the 10–15 ml serum on ice. Add slowly over 1 min with constant stirring. After 15–60 min on ice, centrifuge for 10 min at 7,000–10,000 rpm at 4°C.

   > The precipitate is allowed to form fully at 0°C for 15–60 min. If the solution of antibody protein is 1 mg/ml or less, precipitation is less efficient; yields may be increased if precipitate formation occurs overnight at 0–4°C.

3. Pour off the supernatant and save. (Just in case!) Wash the pellet by resuspending in 50% SAS and disrupting either with a glass stir rod or by drawing the suspension into and out of a pasteur pipet repeatedly. (The volume of 50% SAS is not critical, but usually is at least 10× the estimated volume of the pellet.) Centrifuge the suspension again to obtain a washed pellet. Discard the supernatant.

4. Dissolve the pellet in about 5 ml 0.05 M phosphate buffer pH 8.0. Dialyze at 4°C against 500 ml phosphate buffer. Change the buffer several times over the next 24 hr.

DAY TWO

5. After dialysis, determine the total volume of the dialyzed sample in a graduated cylinder. Check conductivity of the dialyzed sample to confirm that the phosphate is 0.05 M.

   > Some particulates may appear after dialysis. These are protein molecules that have become irreversibly denatured and insoluble.

6. Determine the protein concentration of the sample by measuring absorbance at 280 nm. Microcentrifuge a 0.5-ml sample to clarify and dilute 0.10 ml of the supernatant 50-fold with 0.05 M phosphate buffer. *Freeze the remaining sample for PAGE and Ouchterlony double diffusion.* Measure the absorbance of the diluted sample at 280 nm and calculate the protein concentration, assuming an extinction coefficient of 1.35 for 1 mg/ml γ globulin at 280 nm.

7. Use this γ globulin preparation as starting material for DEAE purification of IgG (Experiment 2-IB).

Questions

1. What is the total mass (in mg) of γ globulin protein obtained by the salt precipitation?

2. What is the percentage yield of γ globulin compared with total protein in the original volume of antiserum (Step 1)?

3. Does the γ globulin preparation contain only anti-glucose oxidase antibody, or does it contain antibodies against other antigens? Explain.

4. IgM class antibody is insoluble in pure water, whereas the other classes of antibody remain soluble. Describe a procedure to isolate IgM independent of the other classes of antibody in serum.

B. DEAE ANION-EXCHANGE CHROMATOGRAPHY

Diethylaminoethyl (DEAE) chromatography is a mild and effective method for separating proteins based on charge. The DEAE group maintains a constant positive charge that is neutralized by a counter ion, usually Cl⁻. Other anions are capable of competing for the positive DEAE group, including proteins that have a net negative charge because of their amino acid composition. For instance, the IgG class of antibodies is somewhat basic, containing slightly more lysine and arginine than glutamate and aspartate residues. Because the isoelectric point of IgG is

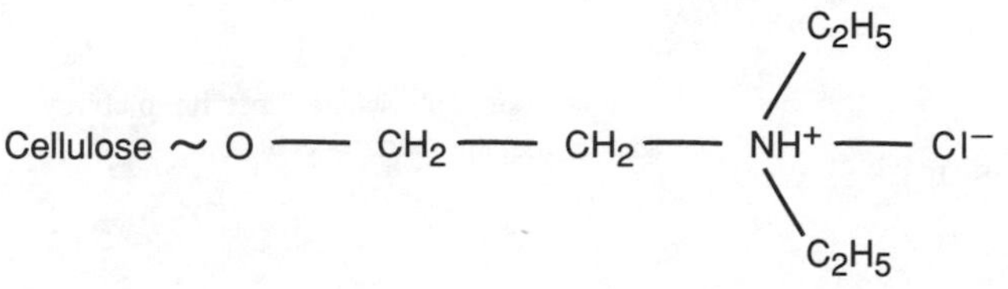

Cellulose $\sim$ O —— CH$_2$ —— CH$_2$ —— NH$^+$ —— Cl$^-$ with C_2H_5 groups above and below the NH$^+$

FIGURE 2.1

DEAE group.

approximately 8, it will not bind to the DEAE group at pH 8. However, other serum proteins with lower pIs (acidic proteins) will be negatively charged and will bind to DEAE. Thus, IgG will be recovered in the "flow through" of the column, leaving the more acidic proteins, including IgM, bound to the DEAE resin (Fahey and Terry, 1986).

Although DEAE is most efficient for purifying IgG, it is also possible to isolate IgM antibody by eluting the DEAE column with increasing concentrations of salt. Phosphate is the classical buffer salt used for immunoglobulin separation by DEAE, but sodium chloride may be used also to increase the salt concentration when buffered with phosphate. Increasing the phosphate from 0.05 to 0.20 M in a linear gradient normally releases the IgM, but yields and purity vary widely, depending on the species of IgM.

Experiment

The γ globulin preparation obtained by ammonium sulfate precipitation will be applied to a column of DEAE–cellulose and fractionated by increasing phosphate concentration. The IgG and IgM fractions will be identified by precipitation in agarose gel (Experiments 4-I,II) and by polyacrylamide electrophoresis (Experiment 2-II).

Materials
□ γ globulin fraction of anti-glucose oxidase (Step 7, Experiment 2-IA)

Immunoglobulins G (IgG) and M (IgM) are the predominant immunoglobulins in serum, at concentrations of approximately 15 and 2 mg/ml, respectively. IgG has a pI of 7.5–8.5, whereas IgM has a pI of 7.0–7.5.

IgM frequently is contaminated with other serum proteins. Additional chromatography on hydroxyapatite (Ca$_5$OH(PO$_4$)$_3$) usually is required to obtain pure IgM (see Bucovsky and Kennett, 1987; Gorbunoff, 1990).

Although the procedure detailed in this experiment is performed at room temperature, protein isolations typically are done at refrigerator temperatures to reduce bacterial growth, protein denaturation, and proteolytic attack.

□ DEAE–cellulose, coarse mesh (Sigma # D 8507)

□ 0.05 M, 0.20 M, and 0.50 M potassium phosphate, pH 8.0

□ 2 × 30-cm glass chromatography column, with scintered glass or glass wool as a resin support

□ 30–40 15-ml capacity test tubes

□ fraction collector (optional)

□ UV spectrophotometer

Use potassium phosphate, since its solubility is greater that the sodium salt at 4°C.

Procedure

DAY ONE

1. Suspend 10 gm DEAE–cellulose, coarse mesh, in approximately 500 ml 0.05 M potassium phosphate, pH 8.0. Allow to swell, with occasional stirring, for 5 min.

2. Adjust pH to 8.0 with 6 N HCl.

3. Allow to settle for 10 min. Pour off the supernatant and any fine particulates (fines) that have not settled.

4. Add fresh buffer to form a slurry of approximately equal volumes of DEAE and buffer; adjust pH to 8 if necessary.

5. Pour a 2.0 × 20-cm column by adding the 50% slurry of DEAE–cellulose to a prepared column while allowing buffer to flow out the bottom. If time permits, run 2–3 column volumes of buffer through the column to complete the equilibration. Allow the buffer to drain until 1 cm buffer remains on top of the column. Either use the column immediately, or store at room temperature with parafilm covering the top of the column.

The DEAE–cellulose used in this experiment is a coarse form of cellulose fiber that allows fast column flow rates, but lowest resolving capacity. Medium and fine celluloses may have more resolving ability, but suffer from substantially slower flow rates. Other DEAEs include microgranular cellulose and Sephadex–DEAE-A50 (Pharmacia), both of which combine good flow rates and high resolving abilities. However, Sephadex–DEAE shrinks with increasing ionic strength, making resin regeneration with high salt washes difficult in the column.

This removal of fines may result in significant loss of resin, but the resultant de-fined resin will have increased flow rates, which may be particularly important in large columns.

This preparation of DEAE–cellulose is abbreviated but suitable for Ig separation. For more precise work, the DEAE may be washed with 0.10 M NaOH for 1–2 min, followed by a thorough washing with water, then 1 M NaCl, and finally the equilibration buffer. Cellulose becomes quite gelatinous in NaOH and must be filtered through two or more layers of filter paper in a Buchner funnel to avoid clogging. Many researchers find this procedure tedious, and use precleaned microgranular DEAE–cellulose or Sephadex–DEAE-A50, which are ready to use out of the bottle, instead.

DAY TWO

PERFORM ALL STEPS AT ROOM TEMPERATURE.

6. Check conductivity and total volume of your dialyzed γ globulin solution, making sure it is 0.05 M potassium phosphate, pH 8.0 (Step 5, Experiment I. A). Apply the globulin preparation to the top of the column. Allow all of it to enter the column, collecting 10-ml fractions. After all the sample has entered the column, follow with 100 ml 0.05 M potassium phosphate, pH 8.0. Monitor the protein elution by reading the absorbance of each fraction at 290 or 300 nm.

7. Continue the elution with 100 ml 0.20 M potassium phosphate, pH 8.0, collecting 10-ml fractions. Finally, elute with 100 ml 0.50 M potassium phosphate, pH 8.0, collecting 10-ml fractions. By increasing the salt concentration in a stepwise fashion, IgG and IgM should be released in separate peaks.

8. For each peak, select the fraction with the highest absorbance and set up two Ouchterlony tests (see Experiment 4-I). The first test will detect the presence of anti-glucose oxidase in the fractions by diffusing against purified glucose oxidase (Experiment 4-I, Format 1). The second test will detect the presence of sheep IgG and IgM in the fractions using commercially available anti-IgG and anti-IgM (Experiment 4-I, Format 2). For this second test, you may want to fill the well 2–3 times with the IgG and IgM fractions (see Step 9).

DAY THREE

9. After 24–48 hr, check the Ouchterlony plates for the presence of precipitin arcs. From these results, determine which DEAE peaks have anti-glucose oxidase antibody and pool the IgG and IgM fractions separately. If the arcs are difficult to see in the plates, you may want to set up the test once again, filling the sample wells 2–3 times, allowing the previous fill to be almost

Prepared columns may be stored at room temperature for several days before bacterial and fungal growth becomes a problem; if in doubt, add sodium azide or thimerosal to 0.01% in the buffers to inhibit growth. Columns stored at 4°C to retard bacterial growth are difficult to warm to room temperature without air escaping and forming bubbles throughout the column. Refrigerating a warm column poses no such problems.

Step elution is less efficient than gradient elution, but is easier to do. A gradient elution reduces "tailing" of an eluting protein peak by releasing the tailing protein with increasing concentration of salt.

Read all fractions at 290 or 300 nm; plot the absorbance of each fraction against the fraction number. The high concentration of protein directly off the column would result in very large absorbance values at a λ_{max} of 280 nm, values too large for the spectrophotometer to read accurately. However, at the wavelengths of 290 or 300 nm, proteins absorb less light, so lower absorbances result.

absorbed by the agar gel. It is often difficult to detect IgM, and you may delete this part of the experiment.

10. Measure the volume and the absorbance at 280 nm of the combined IgG fractions. Calculate the concentration and total IgG protein using an extinction coefficient of 1.35 for a 1 mg/ml solution of IgG at 280 nm. Determine the percentage recovery of the IgG from (a) the original antiserum sample (Step 1, p. 17) and (b) the γ globulin obtained after ammonium sulfate precipitation (Step 5, p. 18).

11. To compare the purity of the IgG, γ globulin, and serum samples, use immunoelectrophoresis (Experiment 4-II) and polyacrylamide gel electrophoresis analysis (Experiment 2-II).

12. To produce F(ab′)$_2$ and Fab fragments from the IgG by pepsin or papain digestion, go to Experiment 2-III.

An extinction coefficient of 1.35 at 280 nm commonly is used to estimate the concentration of immunoglobulin. IgGs have coefficients equal to 1.4 whereas the coefficients IgMs are closer to 1.2 (see Kirschenbaum, 1978). Since the immunoglobulin preparation is impure at this point, any concentration value based on these extinction coefficients is only an approximation of protein concentration. For more accurate protein determinations, use a chemical protein assay.

II. PAGE Analysis of IgG Subunit Structure

Polyacrylamide gel electrophoresis (PAGE), has become the standard method by which to examine the molecular weight, the subunit structure, and the purity of proteins. In this section of the experiment, the various fractions collected during the purification of anti-glucose oxidase IgG will be analyzed by PAGE. Because PAGE is so versatile in the study of both antibodies and antigens, a discussion of the technique will be presented first.

Proteins Are Charged Molecules

Proteins are amphoteric molecules containing both negative carboxyl groups and positive amino groups. The isoelectric point, pI, is the pH at which a protein has no net charge. It is a measure of the sum of the positive and negative groups on a protein and is a convenient way to compare the relative net charges of proteins. Since individual proteins have characteristic pIs, they will migrate at different speeds in response to an electric field.

Polyacrylamide Matrix

During PAGE, proteins are separated as they migrate through a three-dimensional matrix in an electric field. The matrix serves two functions. It separates the proteins according to size, shape, and net charge, and it maintains a constant buffered pH to insure consistent protein charge.

Polyacrylamide is the matrix of choice for protein separation in the 5,00–250,000 molecular weight range. Pores are produced in the matrix by cross-linking linear polyacrylamide chains with bis-acrylamide. The pore size of a polyacrylamide gel may be reduced by increasing the total percentage of acrylamide, % T, or by increasing the degree of cross-linking, % C, with bisacrylamide. In practice, 5% C results in the smallest pores at any given % T. The appropriate % T also must be chosen to produce the correct sized pores to sieve the proteins of interest effectively. Too high a % T will impede movement of proteins into the gel, whereas too low a %T will allow proteins to migrate quickly through the gel with little separation according to protein size. Initiation of free-radical polymerization usually is accomplished by ammonium persulfate and catalyzed by N,N,N',N'-tctramethylethylenediamine (TEMED) (Figure 2.2).

Agarose, a matrix with a more open structure, is most suitable for molecular weight separation of larger molecules such as DNA.

Riboflavin may be used instead of ammonium persulfate to generate free radicals if illuminated by long wavelength ultraviolet light. This method is used if the ammonium persulfate affects the proteins or if extremely low ionic strength is necessary.

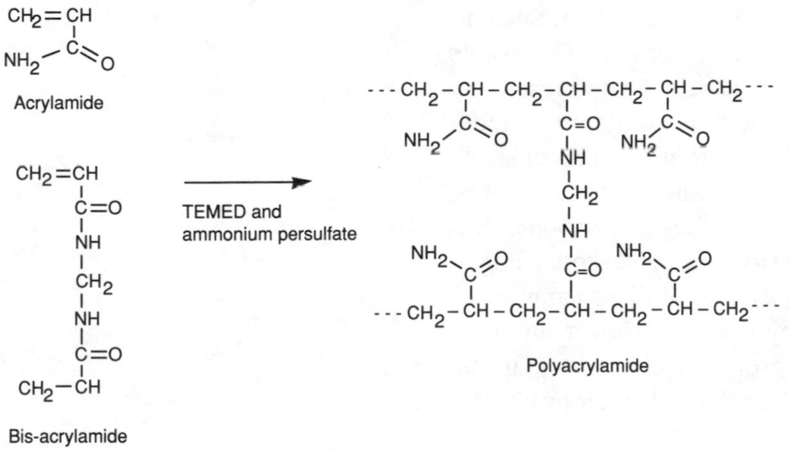

FIGURE 2.2

Representation of the polyacrylamide matrix formed by free-radical initiation.

Electrophoretic Theory

The effect of voltage (E), current (I), resistance (R), and power (P) must be considered when analyzing protein migration during electrophoresis. During electrophoresis, a gel may be considered a resistance through which a protein migrates with a velocity proportional to the current. The resistance of the gel increases over time due to accelerating solute molecules that meet resistance from a number of sources: the matrix, the counter ions, and the viscosity of the solvent. Heat is generated during the run and is proportional to the power. With these considerations in mind, and the three basic electrical equations listed, the effect of I, E, and P on protein movement in electrophoresis can be determined.

> velocity is proportional to I
>
> heat is proportional to P
>
> $I = E/R$
>
> $P = I^2R$
>
> $P = EI$

During electrophoresis, the voltage, current, or power is kept constant. Since R increases during electrophoresis, the effect of maintaining constant E, I, or P varies according to the equations listed. If E is constant, the velocity decreases and the heat generated is constant. If I is constant, the velocity is constant but additional heat is generated. If P is constant, the velocity decreases but heat is constant. Perhaps the most important parameter over which to maintain careful control is heating. Excessive heating of the gel will cause not only increased diffusion of the protein bands, but also inconsistent protein migration from the center to the edges of the gel ("smiling" of the protein bands). Thus, adjustment of these parameters allows a quick run with potential problems caused by heat or a slower run with maximum reliability. Consequently, effective cooling of the gel is important to reduce artifacts in any situation. Heat dissipation can be achieved either by chilled buffers or by chilled support platforms.

Native or Nondenaturing PAGE

In native PAGE, proteins are separated in a nondenaturing buffer according to their net charge (pI important) and effective size in solution (Davis, 1964; Ornstein, 1964). The proteins maintain their native three-dimensional shape as they migrate through the gel. Normally, the gels are run at pH 8–9, at which most proteins have a net negative charge and migrate toward the anode (most proteins have pIs less than 8.0)(Figure 2.3). Of course, if a protein has a pI above 9, it runs toward the cathode, off the gel! The effective size of a protein molecule depends on its molecular weight, the amount of hydration, and its shape (long, flat, spherical). Thus, it is difficult to predict accurately the pattern of migration of a series of proteins through a native gel. Generally, native PAGE is used only when proteins of similar molecular weights must be separated according to charge, or if native structure must be maintained for subsequent function.

SDS–PAGE

In SDS–PAGE, proteins are electrophoresed in the presence of the ionic detergent sodium dodecyl sulfate (SDS). This detergent binds both to the hydrophobic residues and to the peptide backbone of proteins, approximately once every two

SDS: CH_3—$(CH_2)_{11}$—O—$SO_3^-Na^+$

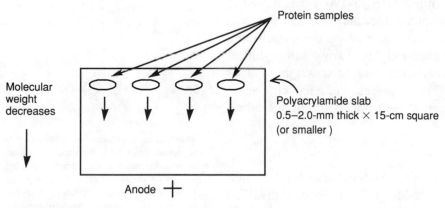

Protein samples

Molecular weight decreases

Polyacrylamide slab
0.5–2.0-mm thick × 15-cm square
(or smaller)

Anode +

FIGURE 2.3

Protein migration in polyacrylamide gel electrophoresis.

amino acids, causing complete unfolding of native protein structure while imparting a constant negative charge per unit length of peptide chain. The proteins assume a random coil shape, roughly a sphere, the size of which depends on the molecular weight of the protein. Thus, SDS-complexed proteins migrate through polyacrylamide at a rate dependent on their molecular weight (Weber and Osborn, 1969). Consequently, SDS–PAGE is used to determine the molecular weights of proteins in a mixture. A plot may be drawn showing a linear relationship between the logarithm of the molecular weight and relative mobility.

Two SDS systems are most common, the continuous system of Weber and Osborn (Weber and Osborn, 1969) and the discontinuous system of Laemmli (Laemmli, 1970). In the continuous system, the protein mixture is layered carefully as a band on top of the separating gel. The thickness of the bands after electrophoresis and, consequently, the resolution of the sample, depends partly on the thickness of the original sample layer. However, in the discontinuous system, the proteins in the sample are compressed by rapidly migrating solvent ions through a porous stacking gel into the separating gel. The proteins are concentrated into a very thin line and are resolved as thin bands (Chrambach et al., 1976).

Subunit Structure of Protein by PAGE and Gel Filtration

Subunit structure of a protein may be examined by SDS–PAGE when used in conjunction with gel filtration. First, the maximum molecular weight of a protein is estimated by gel filtration under mild conditions, under which any subunits of a protein are bound together. Second, the molecular weights of any disulfide-linked subunits are determined by SDS–PAGE. Finally, the molecular weight of individual subunits is determined by SDS–PAGE in the presence of a reducing agent that breaks disulfide bonds, for example, 2-mercaptoethanol (2-ME) or dithiothreitol (DTT)(Figure 2.4).

Sample Preparation and Staining

Samples normally are treated prior to PAGE with 1% SDS in buffer for 2–10 min at 100°C or 60 min at 37°C. A reducing agent (2-ME, DTT) is added if disulfide bonds are to be broken; urea (3–5 M) is included with samples that are extremely insoluble in aqueous solutions. High concentrations of NaCl and $(NH_4)_2SO_4$ cause

Determination of protein molecular weight by SDS–PAGE is reasonably accurate to ±5%, but may be affected by unusual amino acid composition or high carbohydrate content. If exact molecular weight must be known, then an amino acid end group determination followed by amino acid analysis or sequencing should be performed. This information will provide the number of peptide chains (end group analysis) and total mass (amino acid analysis) of the sample, from which molecular weight may be calculated.

After sample treatment, any free sulfhydryls may be alkylated with a 1.1 molar excess of iodoacetamide or iodoacetic acid over reducing agent. This stops reformation of disulfides during electrophoresis. In practice, alkylation is seldom done, since the excessive amount of reducing agent in the sample is usually adequate to inhibit disulfide formation.

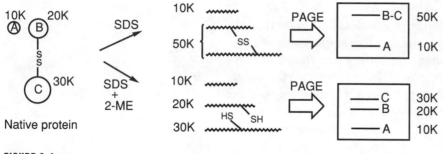

FIGURE 2.4

SDS–PAGE on a multisubunit protein. The A subunit is bound noncovalently to B and C which are disulfide bonded to each other.

precipitation of the SDS as the sodium or ammonium salt, and must be removed by dialysis or on desalting columns before SDS addition. After SDS treatment, samples may be stored at −20°C for months.

After electrophoresis, gels normally are analyzed with protein stains. The two most popular staining reagents are Coomassie blue dye, detecting 1–10 μg protein per band, and silver reduction, detecting 10–100 ng per band (Appendix C). No matter how pure a protein is believed to be, when a large amount is electrophoresed and a sensitive stain is used, other bands will appear. Also, caution is in order when equating protein staining intensities to relative concentrations, since different proteins absorb dyes or silver to varying degrees. Staining procedures are also available to detect carbohydrate on proteins (Appendix C).

Radioactive proteins also may be detected after separation by electrophoresis. For this procedure, the slab gel is most effective and first is dried onto paper or between sheets of cellophane. The dried gel then is placed next to X-ray film in a light-tight box, and stored at freezer temperatures for hours or days. The radioactive emissions expose the photographic X-ray emulsion, while the cool temperature reduces background fog. After development, the film shows dark bands corresponding to any radioactive protein.

Staining for carbohydrate may be done either directly on the gels (fluorescent stain) or after transfer of proteins to blotting membrane (peroxidase stain) (Appendix C).

Gradient Gels

Occasionally, the proteins in a mixture span too large a molecular weight range to be separated effectively with a "linear" gel containing a fixed percentage of acrylamide. To separate these mixtures, a gel with an increasing percentage of acrylamide toward the anode, a gradient gel, is employed. These gels retard the migration of low molecular weight components, allowing better separation. Further, the proteins tend to migrate in narrower bands. They migrate into increasing percentages of acrylamide, slowing the leading edge and allowing the trailing edge of the band to catch up.

Experiment

In this procedure, you will analyze partially pure fractions of anti-glucose oxidase IgG obtained during ammonium sulfate precipitation and DEAE chromatography. Samples will be subjected to SDS–PAGE and stained with either Coomassie dye or silver to visualize the protein bands.

Materials

- □ reagents for preparing and staining PAGE gels (Appendix C)
- □ slab gel electrophoresis apparatus (e.g. Mini-PROTEAN II, BioRad #165-2940)
- □ refrigerator or cold room to cool electrophoresis during run (optional)
- □ power supply, 200 V, 100 mA minimum
- □ samples of anti-glucose oxidase at various stages of purity:
    anti-glucose oxidase serum (Step 1, p. 17)
    50 % SAS dilution (Step 6, p. 18)
    DEAE purified IgG (Step 10, p. 22)
- □ 10 × 75-mm glass test tubes or 1.5-ml microfuge tubes
- □ boiling water bath
- □ 10–20 μl adjustable micropipets or Hamilton syringes

Procedure

The procedure below requires 4 hr, and usually more, when the reagents have been prepared earlier. The time may be shortened if the running gel is poured beforehand (stored at 4°C) and the stacking gel is poured at the beginning of the procedure.

1. *Prepare PAGE gels*. This takes up to 2 hr, so start early. The reagents and procedures for the PAGE gels are included in Appendix C. Be careful with the acrylamide solutions, since monomeric acrylamide is a neurotoxin; wear gloves and rinse out glassware soon after use.

2. *Dilute samples for PAGE*. First, choose the samples to be electrophoresed (See step 4). Then, during the polymerization of the gels, dilute your samples. Each sample will be loaded onto the gel in a volume of 5–20 µl, and should contain at least 5 µg protein. Thus, the protein samples should be at concentrations of 250–1000 µg/ml. Dilute any concentrated samples to this concentration range with an appropriate low-sodium buffer such as phosphate buffered saline (PBS) or 1× sample preparation buffer (see Step 3).

3. *Treat samples with sample preparation buffer (SPB)*. Some of the samples will require a reducing SPB to break disulfide bonds and others a nonreducing SPB (See Table 2.1). SPB is a 4× stock solution and should be diluted with your sample to obtain 1× SPB. For example, pipette 100 µl protein into a small tube (10 × 75-mm glass test tube or a 1.5-ml microfuge tube) and add 33 µl 4× SPB. Seal with parafilm or snap cap, prick a small hole in the top with a 23- or 25-gauge needle, and incubate at 37°C for 30 min or 95°C (boiling water) for 5 min. Remove samples from heat and cool to room temperature.

4. Pipette 5–20 µl of each sample into the appropriate wells. A suggested placement in the gel is shown in Table 2.1. Remember the order and orientation of the gel in the electrophoresis apparatus. Electrophorese at 4°C until the *m*-cresol purple dye starts to emerge from the bottom of the gel. This should take about 90 min at 100 V for a minigel.

TABLE 2.1

Treatment and Placement of Samples

SPB	Lane	Sample
Reduced	1	standard molecular weight proteins
	2	DEAE-purified anti-glucose oxidase IgG
	3	50% SAS γ globulin anti-glucose oxidase
	4	anti-glucose oxidase serum
	5	blank well
Nonreduced	6	standard molecular weight proteins
	7	DEAE-purified anti-glucose oxidase IgG
	8	50% SAS γ globulin anti-glucose oxidase
	9	anti-glucose oxidase serum
	10	blank well

5. Separate the gel from the glass plates, scrape away the stacking gel, and immerse the separating gel in the Coomassie dye. Allow to stain for at least 2 hr with gentle agitation; overnight staining is acceptable. Destain with 3–4 changes of destaining solution, allowing 30–60 min of gentle agitation between each change.

DAY TWO

6. Place the gel on a glass plate, and measure the distance each band migrated from the top of the gel. For the standard proteins, plot these distances against the logarithm of the molecular weight on graph paper. This is a standard molecular weight graph. Determine the molecular weight of the sample bands from the standard graph by extrapolation.

7. If desired, dry the gel between cellophane sheets (Appendix C) or photograph for a permanent record.

III. Fragmentation of IgG by Partial Proteolysis

Immunoglobulin IgG molecules are Y-shaped proteins composed of two heavy, H, and two light, L, peptide chains. A hinge region between the C_{H_1} and C_{H_2} domains is susceptible to proteolytic attack by enzymes such as papain and pepsin, resulting in fragmentation of the IgG. The Fab and $F(ab')_2$ fragments contain the entire L chain, disulfide linked to a portion of the H chain (V_c and C_{H_1} domains). The Fc fragment contains the remaining portion of the two H chains (C_{H_2} and C_{H_3}), disulfide linked together (Figure 2.5).

The Fab and Fc fragments have been pivotal in elucidating the structure of immunoglobulins (Porter, 1959) and are useful in many immunological tech-niques. The Fab fragment is univalent, so it binds antigen without cross-linking or precipitation of antigen. It also does not promote patching or capping when bound to cell surface antigens. The $F(ab')_2$ fragment is divalent and may cross-link antigens. However, both fragments lack the Fc region and may be useful when effector functions, such as complement fixation or binding to cellular Fc receptors, are not desired. Thus, Fab and $F(ab')_2$ may exhibit both reduced

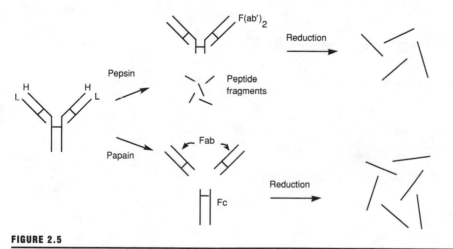

FIGURE 2.5

Pepsin and papain fragmentation of IgG.

nonspecific binding in immunoassays and greater tissue permeation compared with whole IgG.

F(ab′)$_2$ fragments usually are prepared by pepsin digestion of IgG, whereas Fab fragments result from papain digestion. The Fc fragments generated by both enzymes normally are not desired and are removed by chromatography (Mage, 1980; Parham *et al.*, 1982). Pepsin is a small protease of MW 35,000 that cleaves IgG into F(ab′)$_2$ fragments and Fc peptides at low pH. The F(ab′)$_2$ fragments are purified from residual IgG and peptides by gel filtration and, if necessary, protein A affinity chromatography. (Protein A will remove IgG by binding to the Fc portion.) Papain, MW 23,000, requires a reduced active site sulfhydryl for activity, and cleaves IgG into Fab and Fc fragments. These fragments usually are resolved by DEAE ion-exchange chromatography, but also may be separated by protein A affinity chromatography.

Experiment

In this experiment, goat or sheep IgG will be digested first by either pepsin or papain, and then analyzed by PAGE. Abbreviated procedures for separation of the resultant fragments are given as the last step in each procedure.

Materials

☐ goat or sheep IgG (γ globulins may be used, depending on purity, and are considerably less expensive than IgG)

☐ pepsin, porcine stomach, crystallized (Sigma #P6887)

☐ PBS (see Appendix B)

☐ 0.20 M sodium acetate, pH 4.3

☐ 1 M potassium phosphate, pH 7.0–7.4

☐ papain (mercuripapain is a more stable form of papain and may be used alternatively; Sigma #P4762 or P9886)

☐ papain buffer, pH 6.8
   25 mM potassium phosphate
   10 mM EDTA

□ cysteine

□ iodoacetamide

□ 37°C incubator or water bath

Procedure

Pepsin digestion

DAY ONE

1. Dissolve 5.0 mg IgG in 1.0 ml 0.20 M acetate, pH 4.3.

2. Add pepsin to 2% by weight relative to the IgG. Since this would be a very small amount to weigh accurately, add the pepsin in the form of a solution. Weigh out 5 mg pepsin and dissolve in 1.0 ml PBS. (At pH 7.0–7.5, pepsin is essentially inactive.) Calculate the volume of this solution needed to provide 2% by weight of pepsin relative to the IgG. Add this volume to the IgG. Cap the tube with an airtight cap.

DAY TWO

3. Allow pepsin to digest IgG at 37°C for 12-18 hr. Remove from incubator and add 50 μl 1 M potassium phosphate, pH 7.4, to achieve 0.050 M phosphate. Finally, adjust the pH to 7.0–7.5 with approximately 25 μl 1 M NaOH. Check with pH paper.

4. Analyze for F(ab')₂ production on reduced and nonreduced PAGE, using a 7.5% gel to insure that the high molecular weight IgG and F(ab')₂ will enter the gel.

Papain digestion

DAY ONE

5. Dissolve 5.0 mg IgG in 1.0 ml papain buffer. Set aside.

6. Incubate a 1 mg/ml solution of papain in papain buffer containing 50 mM cysteine for 15 min at 37°C. Cysteine maintains the single sulfhydryl in papain in an active state.

Time, pH, acetate concentration, age of pepsin and IgG, and species of IgG have a great effect on the cleavage and production of active F(ab')₂ fragments. The conditions given in this experiment should be considered approximate, and may be changed to produce optimum yields. The pH is perhaps the most critical of the variables. Values between 3.2 and 3.5 may require only a 1-hr incubation with 1% pepsin to produce complete cleavage, whereas values between 4.7 and 5.0 may require 5–6% pepsin for significant cleavage within 18 hr. For best results, remove aliquots at 30 min, and 1, 3, 6, and 18 hr (followed by neutralization to pH 7) and run all these samples on PAGE to determine optimal incubation time. Goat IgG should be digested starting at pH 4.3, 0.2 M acetate; it tends to be digested more quickly than rabbit IgG.

If the F(ab') fragments are to be used for further experimentation, they may be purified by conventional gel filtration (Sephadex G-150 or Sephacryl S-200) or HPLC (TSK G3000 SW). This removes pepsin and peptides, but may result in slight contamination by whole IgG. Protein-A chromatography will remove any remaining IgG. The purification is not difficult, but is time consuming (see Mage, 1980).

7. Add papain to 1% by weight relative to IgG and incubate for 1 hr at 37°C. To facilitate addition of a small amount of papain, dissolve papain separately to 1–2 mg/ml and add to the IgG in liquid form to achieve the 1% weight per weight IgG.

8. Add iodoacetamide to 30 mM (5.5 mg/ml) to inactivate the papain by acylation of the active-site sulfhydryl. Papain will remain active if iodoacetamide is not added, and may continue cleaving even in the SDS sample preparation buffer used for PAGE.

9. Analyze Fab fragment production on reduced and nonreduced PAGE. Use a 10% gel to separate any residual IgG from the Fab and Fc fragments most effectively.

DAY TWO

10. If desired, separate Fab from Fc and IgG by DEAE chromatography. The strength of binding to DEAE increases from Fab to IgG to Fc. The incubation mixture is dialyzed against 5 mM phosphate, pH 7.5, and applied to a DEAE column equilibrated in the same buffer. The Fab is eluted with the starting buffer, followed by a 0.0 to 0.2 M NaCl gradient elution of a small amount of residual IgG and Fc.

Immunoelectrophoresis of the Fab and Fc fragments should show an arc of Fc anionic to that of Fab when developed with anti-whole IgG. A reaction of nonidentity should be seen between the two different fragments on Ouchterlony double diffusion also when developed with anti-whole IgG.

REFERENCES

Bukovsky, J., and Kennett, R. H. (1987). Simple and rapid purification of monoclonal antibodies from cell culture supernatants and ascites fluids by hydroxyapatite chromatography on analytical and preparative scales. *Hybridoma* **6,** 219–228.

Chrambach, A., Jovin, T. M., Svedsen, P. J., and Rodbard, D. (1976). Analytical and preparative polyacrylamide gel electrophoresis. An objectively defined fractionation route, apparatus, and procedures. *In* "Methods of Protein Separation" (N. Catsimpoolas, ed.), Vol. 2, pp. 27–144. Plenum, New York.

Davis, B. J. (1964). Disc electrophoresis - II: Methods and applications to human serum proteins. *Ann. N. Y. Acad. Sci.* **121**, 404–427.

Dawson, R. M. C., Elliott, D. C., Elliott, W. H., and Jones, K. M. (1986). *"Data for Biochemical Research,"* 3d Ed. Oxford Science Publications, Oxford.

England, S., and Seifter, S. (1990). Precipitation techniques. *Meth. Enzymol.* **182**, 285–300.

Fahey, J. L., and Terry, E. W. (1986). Ion exchange chromatography and gel filtration. *In "Handbook of Experimental Immunology"* (D. M. Weir, ed.), pp. 8.1–8.6. Blackwell Scientific, Oxford.

Gorbunoff, M. J. (1990). Protein chromatography on hydroxyapatite columns. *Meth. Enzymol.* **182,** 329–339.

Ingham, K. C. (1990). Precipitation of proteins with polyethylene glycol. *Meth. Enzymol.* **182**, 301–306.

Kirschenbaum, D. M. (1978). Molar absorptivity values for proteins at selected wavelengths of the UV and visible region, XV. *Anal. Biochem.* **87**, 223–242.

Laemmli, U. K. (1970). Cleavage of structural proteins during the assembly of the head of bacteriophage T4. *Nature (London)* **227**, 680–685.

Mage, M. G. (1980). Preparation of Fab fragments from IgGs of different animal species. *Meth. Enzymol.* **70**, 142–150.

Ornstein, L. (1964). Disc electrophoresis-I: Background and theory. *Ann. N. Y. Acad. Sci.* **121**, 321–349.

Parham, P., Androlewicz, M. J., Brodsky, F. M., Holmes, N. J. and Ways, J. P. (1982). Monoclonal antibodies: purification, fragmentation and application to structural and functional studies of class I MHC antigens. *J. Immunol. Methods* **53**, R101–141.

Porter, R. R. (1959). The hydrolysis of rabbit γ-globulin and antibody with crystalline papain. *Biochem. J.* **73,** 119.

Stoscheck, C. M. (1990). Quantitation of protein. *Meth. Enzymol.,* **182,** 50–68.

Weber, K., and Osborn, M. (1969). The reliability of molecular weight determinations by dodecyl sulfate–polyacrylamide gel electrophoresis. *J. Biol. Chem.* **224,** 4406–4412.

Quantitative Precipitin Curve

Background Information

Serum from an immunized animal will contain both specific antibodies to the immunizing antigen and nonspecific antibodies to a wide variety of antigens the animal has encountered over its lifetime. To determine the concentration of specific antibodies in serum, the ability of the antibodies to bind antigen must be used. It is impossible to determine specific antibodies by techniques that measure total antibody only. This experiment shows how to determine both the concentration of specific antibody in serum and the number of epitopes on an antigen.

Antigens

An antigen is a substance capable of binding to antibody molecules or immune-system cell antigen receptors. Although a wide variety of organic molecules may be antigens, most naturally occurring biological antigens are either soluble or membrane-bound proteins or polysaccharides. Antibodies elicited against an antigen bind small defined areas called *antigenic determinants* or epitopes. Typically, a protein antigen will have 3–6 epitopes, each consisting of 3–15 amino acids (Davies *et al.*, 1988), whereas a polysaccharide epitope will consist of 1–4 sugar monomers (Kabat, 1976). For protein antigens, an epitope may be formed from amino acids in a linear sequence (a linear epitope) or from distal parts of the protein chain that fold in a local area (a conformational or discontinuous epitope) (Figure 3.1). Most single-chain proteins have only one copy of each epitope, but proteins consisting of identical subunits will have identical epitopes on each subunit. Antigens containing two or more epitopes, identical or different, are termed *polyvalent*.

Binding of an antibody to an antigen occurs by hydrogen bonding, ionic interactions, hydrophobic interactions, and van der Waals attractions.

Although only the exterior epitopes of a protein are exposed to the solvent, and presumably to the antibody, the interior epitopes also may be antigenic. Apparently, proteins are broken into smaller peptides by cells of the immune system; these peptides also may be presented as antigens. Thus, antibodies may not recognize interior epitopes in native proteins, but may recognize them if the protein is denatured. This concept is especially useful for the generation of vaccines, in which masked epitopes on pathogenic organisms are often effective immunizing agents. Further, interior and exterior epitopes may be equally important when detecting denatured antigens with antibody.

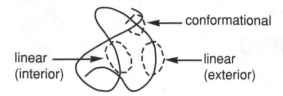

FIGURE 3.1

Conformational and linear epitopes on a protein.

Polyclonal and Monoclonal Antibodies

An immunized animal usually produces a polyclonal antiserum against a protein antigen. The antiserum will contain a heterogeneous pool of antibodies, each specific for a different epitope on the antigen. Each different antibody type results from a *clone* of antibody-producing plasma cells, hence the term polyclonal. The heterogeneity in polyclonal antiserum arises for several different reasons. First, different animals will elicit a different pool of clones, producing a unique polyclonal antiserum. Second, as the immunization period continues, different subclasses of antibodies arise: IgM antibodies are prevalent early in the immune response whereas IgGs arise later. Finally, as the immune response matures, the binding constants between antibody and antigen often increase (Klinman and Press, 1975). The heterogeneous nature of polyclonal antiserum is often its strength; mature polyclonal antiserum binds antigens strongly, and is very useful in a wide range of antibody-based immunoassays.

In contrast, monoclonal antibodies result from the stimulation of a single clone of antibody-producing cells. A monoclonal antibody is one molecular species capable of binding only one epitope on an antigen. Although monoclonal antibodies do arise spontaneously in nature during certain neoplasms of the lymphocytes, usually they are produced deliberately from *in vitro* fusion of myeloma cells and an antibody-producing lymphocyte. The resulting *fusoma* or hybridoma is an immortal cell line capable of producing one specific antibody in large quantities. These cells may be frozen for many years, potentially offering an endless supply of the antibody-producing cells. Although monoclonal antibody preparations are homogeneous and are highly specific in their binding, they may not be as useful as

A myeloma cell is a neoplastic plasma cell, a *plasmacytoma*, that may be grown indefinitely in tissue culture as an immortal cell line.

polyclonal antibody preparation in many techniques that require cross-linking or precipitation of antigen molecules. However, their exquisite specificity and homogeneity may be preferred in more refined structural techniques and in therapeutic applications. Further, monoclonal antibody may be elicited against antigens that are impossible to purify; the impure antigen induces many clones that are selected at a later step to produce an antigen-specific hybridoma.

Precipitation Curve

Addition of antibody to a sample of polyvalent antigen may result in antigen–antibody complexes large enough to precipitate out of solution. The formation of a precipitate is a hallmark of an antigen–antibody reaction and is used in a number of assays that detect the presence of either antigen or antibody. The degree of precipitation varies with the ratio of antigen to antibody. If a constant amount of antibody is mixed with increasing amounts of antigen, the precipitation will increase to a maximum and then decrease. Maximal precipitation occurs when all the antigen and all the antibody are incorporated into a lattice, usually when 2–4 antibodies bind to one antigen (Zone B, Figure 3.2). When either antigen or antibody is in excess, smaller antigen–antibody complexes form, resulting in decreased precipitation (Zones A and C, Figure 3.2). It is important to understand that precipitation occurs only if the antigen is polyvalent. If an antigen has only one epitope, it cannot bind two antibodies simultaneously to form a lattice.

The quantitative precipitin curve yields two types of information: the amount of specific antibody in the serum and the average number of functional epitopes on the antigen molecule. To determine the amount of antibody, the precipitate is obtained by centrifugation and quantitated by spectrophotometry. The amount of antigen used in the assay then is subtracted; the amount of antibody is the resulting difference. The number of epitopes on the antigen then may be estimated from the molar ratio of antibody to antigen in the precipitate.

Experiment

In this experiment, the concentration of anti-glucose oxidase antibody in an immune serum will be determined by precipitation with the antigen. In addition, the number of antigenic determinants or epitopes on glucose oxidase will be estimated.

A monoclonal antibody preparation can form a precipitate only if the antigen has two or more identical epitopes. This might occur if the antigen is composed of two or more identical subunits, or if the antigen is highly conserved and has several repeating sequences. However, most single subunit proteins have no duplication of their sequences that would provide two identical epitopes on one protein chain. Thus, polyclonal antisera, which contain antibodies to many different epitopes on one antigen, normally are better precipitating antisera than monoclonal antibody preparations.

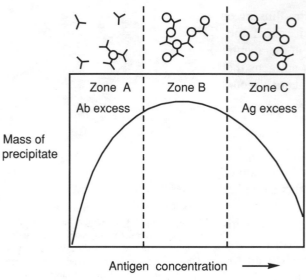

FIGURE 3.2

Antigen-antibody precipitin curve. Ab, antibody; Ag, antigen.

Materials

- ☐ glucose oxidase (GO), 2 mg/ml
- ☐ anti-glucose oxidase antiserum, produced in any species
- ☐ 0.10 M NaOH
- ☐ PBS (Appendix B)
- ☐ microfuge tubes
- ☐ 37°C water bath
- ☐ UV spectrophotometer

Procedure

DAY ONE

1. Fill eight 1.5-ml, microfuge tubes with both glucose oxidase and PBS buffer according to table 1. Label the tops of the microfuge tubes so the numbers won't be rubbed off the sides of the tubes during the subsequent steps.

2. Add 200 µl anti-glucose oxidase serum to each tube, mix gently, and incubate at 37°C for 30 min, followed by 0°C for 10 min. Mix gently every 5 min. Tubes may be stored at 4°C for several days if necessary.

DAY TWO

3. Microfuge tubes for 1 min, remove supernatants by aspiration with a pasteur pipet, and resuspend the pellet with approximately 1 ml PBS. Centrifuge again and remove supernatants. This process is called washing the precipitate. Repeat washing once again, and remove as much of the buffer as possible without disturbing the pellet.

4. Dissolve the washed pellets by adding 1.0 ml of 0.10 M NaOH to each tube.

5. Quantitatively transfer the contents of each microfuge tube to separate glass test tubes, each containing 1.0 ml 0.1 M NaOH.

6. Zero the spectrophotometer at 280 nm with 0.1 M NaOH. Then, read the absorbance for each test tube from Step 5. Subtract the absorbance of anti-serum-blank Tube 1 from that of all other tubes.

Note that 500 µl constant volume is maintained in all tubes.

NaOH denatures all protein structure, releasing the antigens and antibody into solution.

The minimum volume for 4-ml cuvets is 2 ml. If smaller volume cuvets are used, 1 ml total volume should be used.

TABLE 1
Preparation of Microfuge Tubes for Precipitation

Solution	Tube no.							
(µl)	1	2	3	4	5	6	7	8
GO	0	25	50	100	150	200	300	400
PBS	500	475	450	400	350	300	200	100

7. Plot the absorbance values (vertical axis) against glucose oxidase (μg) (horizontal axis). This is a quantitative precipitin curve.

8. Determine the anti-glucose oxidase antibody content of the serum in mg/ml. To do this, first identify the tube containing the maximum precipitate from the graph. Assume all the added anti-glucose oxidase antibody and all the glucose oxidase are precipitated in this tube. Second, calculate the expected absorbance if all the precipitated glucose oxidase from this tube was in the 2 ml in Step 5. Use an extinction coefficient of 1.68 for a 1 mg/ml solution of glucose oxidase at 280 nm. Third, determine the difference between this calculated absorbance and the actual absorbance measured in Step 6. *This difference is due to the anti-glucose oxidase in the test tube.* Fourth, with this difference value, calculate the anti-glucose oxidase concentration using an extinction coefficient of 1.5 for a 1 mg/ml solution at 280 nm. Finally, calculate the concentration of anti-glucose oxidase in the serum using the appropriate dilution corrections.

It is possible to assay for free antigen and antibody in the supernatant to verify that both are precipitated completely. For instance, if ^{125}I-labeled glucose oxidase were incorporated into this experiment, the amount of antigen precipitated could be determined precisely rather than estimated.

This extinction value is higher than the 1.35 used for IgG in neutral solutions. The 0.1 M NaOH causes an increase in absorbance, probably by uncovering some aromatic amino acid residues normally sequestered inside the immunoglobulin molecule.

9. Calculate the average number of epitopes on the glucose oxidase molecule identified with this serum. Start by calculating the concentration of both antigen (glucose oxidase) and antibody in each of the precipitin curve tubes, as done in Step 8. Next, convert the concentrations of antigen and antibody to molar values; use 80,000 and 150,000 gm/mol for the molecular weights of the glucose oxidase and antibody, respectively. Then, calculate the molar ratio of antibody to antigen for each tube. Plot this ratio (vertical axis) against antigen added (horizontal axis) and extrapolate the maximum antibody:antigen ratio when the antigen concentration is 0. At this limit, the antibody is in infinite excess over antigen and should be saturating the epitopes on the antigen.

This extrapolated value for epitopes is not meant to be the absolute number possible on the antigen, but only the functional number for the antigen–antibody system being tested.

Questions

1. What is the average molecular weight of one glucose oxidase molecule and its associated antibodies at maximum precipitation? Is this molecular weight large enough to explain the precipitation seen? (Proteins with molecular weights of up to 1×10^6 normally are soluble.)

2. Do both binding sites on one antibody bind to the same glucose oxidase molecule? Remember, glucose oxidase is a single subunit protein.

3. Would you expect a monoclonal anti-glucose oxidase to yield a precipitin curve similar to that of the polyclonal antiserum? Why?

REFERENCES

Davies, D. R., Sheriff, S., and Padlan, E. A. (1988). Antibody–antigen complexes. *J. Biol. Sci.* **263,** 10541–10544.

Kabat, E. A. (1976). *"Structural Concepts in Immunology and Immunochemistry," 2d Ed.* Holt, Rinehart, and Winston, New York.

Klinman, N. R., and Press, J. (1975). The B cell specificity repertoire: Its relationship to definable subpopulations. *Transplant. Rev.* **24,** 41–83.

Precipitation Analysis in Gel

In this section, three immunoprecipitation techniques will be presented that are used to detect the presence of antibodies or antigens. Although all are similar in their use of immune precipitation in a gel matrix, they vary in their application. Briefly, Ouchterlony double diffusion is the most widely used research gel technique for the detection of antibody or antigen, whereas immunoelectrophoresis and radial immunodiffusion are the most widely used clinical gel techniques for the detection of suspect antigens (Clausen, 1977; Ouchterlony and Nilsson, 1986). The techniques are discussed separately, each discussion giving an overview of the technique followed by an experimental section.

I. Ouchterlony Double Diffusion

Double diffusion in agar gels is a semiquantitative technique to determine antibody (Ab) and antigen (Ag) specificity. It is neither sophisticated nor sensitive compared with other modern immunochemical techniques, but remains popular because it is dependable and easy to perform. The technique is useful in assaying antibody production in an animal, in following the purification of an antigen, and in measuring cross-reactivity of similar antigens.

If samples of Ab and Ag are placed in two separate wells in an agar gel, the Ab and Ag slowly diffuse radially from each well. The agar is an inert support matrix that allows slow diffusion of both samples. When the Ab and Ag meet, a specific Ab–Ag complex forms that is visible as a white precipitin line between the wells. The agar normally has a pH of 8, at which immunoglobulins have little net charge. This pH favors specific Ab–Ag precipitation because the

Agar is extracted from seaweed and consists of two linear polysaccharides, agarose and agaropectin. Both of these polysaccharides are composed primarily of 1→3 linked galactose, but agaropectin contains up to 4% negatively charged sulfate groups whereas agarose is neutral. Agar dissolves in boiling water and forms a stable gel on cooling to 35–40°C.

immunoglobulins show both the least nonspecific ionic interaction with the antigen and the least repulsive forces among themselves.

If two similar antigens in different wells diffuse toward an antibody, a precipitate pattern may form containing "spurs." The spurs are overlapping precipitin lines and often provide information about similarities between antigens. In Figure 4.1, antigen A and antigen B share common determinants, but antigen A has additional determinants that react with the antiserum forming a spur over B. Antigens C and B may share common determinants, but both have additional determinants that differ, causing the overlapping spurs.

When using whole antiserum as the source of antibody, the precipitin bands formed in double diffusion are enhanced by the binding of other serum proteins to the precipitate. Chief among these are the C3 and C4 proteins from the complement cascade system. Purified IgG fractions of antibody or affinity-purified antibodies often show considerably weaker precipitin lines because of the absence of these complement components.

The distance from the Ab and Ag wells at which the precipitin line forms is a rough estimation of the concentration of Ab and Ag. The closer the line is to a well, the less concentrated the sample in the well is. This information is often useful when testing for relative concentrations of Ab or Ag, but is not useful for absolute concentration. The sensitivity of immunodiffusion is limited by the ability of a visible precipitin line to be formed; if closely spaced wells are used, 1–5 µg Ag may be detected.

Experiment

In this experiment, you will test the fractions of anti-glucose oxidase purified in Experiment 2 by two different gel formats. In the first format, the presence of anti-

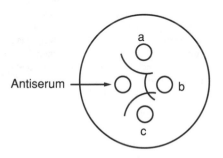
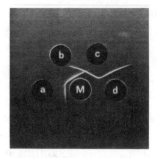

FIGURE 4.1

Spur formation in Ouchterlony double diffusion. M, antiserum to human serum; a, human IgA; b, human IgG; c, human albumin; d, antiserum to human albumin.

glucose oxidase antibody will be determined by using glucose oxidase antigen in a round gel plate. In the second format, anti-glucose oxidase raised in a goat will serve as the antigen and will be detected by using anti-goat IgG antibody on a microscope slide gel plate.

Anti-glucose oxidase	Glucose oxidase	Anti-glucose oxidase	Anti-IgG
(Ab)	(Ag)	(Ag)	(Ab)

Format 1   Format 2

Materials

□ samples of anti-glucose oxidase raised in a goat (or sheep or rabbit) at various stages of purity:

Format 1   anti-glucose oxidase serum (Step 1, Experiment 2,I,A
     50% SAS γ globulin (Step 6, Experiment 2,I,A
     DEAE purified IgG (Step 9, Experiment 2,I,B

Format 2   fractions off DEAE column (Steps 6 and 7, Experiment 2,I,B

□ anti-goat (or sheep or rabbit) IgG and anti-goat (or sheep or rabbit) IgM, both raised in a species different from the one used to raise the primary antibody.

□ 60-mm and 100-mm plastic disposable Petri dishes

□ microscope slides

□ buffer composed of 0.15 M NaCl, 0.01 M Tris, pH 7.5–8.0, 0.005 M EDTA, 0.02% NaN_3

□ agar or agarose

□ 3–4-mm cork borer

□ two single-edged razor blades taped together, to form a double-edged "knife"

□ blunt-tipped 16-gauge needle, connected to a water aspirator with flexible tubing

□ hot plate

□ 50–60°C water bath

Anti-IgG and anti-IgM sera are normally heavy chain specific, that is, the antisera have been absorbed to remove any antibodies specific for light chains, leaving only antibodies that bind to the heavy chains in the IgG or IgM molecule. These antisera also are referred to as "Fc specific" or "H chain specific." Antibodies to the light chain isotypes, kappa (κ) and lambda (λ), will bind to *all* the Ig classes to some degree, since all classes share the same κ and λ light chains.

Procedure

Format 1: Preparation of round gel plate to detect presence of anti-glucose
        oxidase

DAY ONE

1. Prepare 100 ml 1% weight per volume (w/v) agarose in the buffer. Heat the suspension slowly to dissolve the agarose. It may have to boil gently to dissolve the agarose fully. (Be careful: boiling agarose solutions scorch, bump, and froth furiously! If possible, use a hot plate with a magnetic stirrer to avoid scorching.) Once dissolved, keep the agarose liquid at 50–60°C in a waterbath for use in Step 2 and Step 7.

2. Pipette 12–13 ml (one full 10-ml disposable pipet) hot agarose into plastic 60-mm diameter Petri dishes. Allow to cool on level bench with lids off. Finally, replace lids and store sealed at 4°C for 2–6 months if not used immediately.

3. Punch a series of holes in an agarose plate with a well-sharpened 3- or 4-mm cork borer. Punch a pentagon pattern using Figure 4.2 as a guide. The distance between wells should be no more than 4–6 mm. Remove the agarose plugs from the holes with a sharp spatula or wooden stick.

4. Fill each well with 50–70 μl of either antibody fractions or glucose oxidase, as shown in Figure 4.2, or use other combinations.

5. Cover the plate and allow to sit 12–24 hr at room temperature; begin checking for precipitin bands after 4–6 hr.

DAY TWO

6. Identify any precipitin bands formed between the center and outer wells. To detect faint bands, illuminate the plate from the side with a desk lamp while looking through the plate against a dark background.

Refill the DEAE pools 2–3 times if possible; purified antibodies tend to produce less visible precipitin bands than whole antisera. Allow the first fill to diffuse into the gel (37°C speeds this process), then apply the next fill, and so on.

To decrease the gradual dissipation of the bands which occurs after several days, store at 4°C. Alternatively, the gels may be stained and dried for storage after first soaking in several changes of saline for 2–3 days followed by water for 2–3 hr. This removes free proteins and salts. The gels are stained with 0.5% amido schwartz in 5% acetic acid in water, destained with 5% acetic acid, and finally allowed to air dry after a 1–2 hr soaking in 1% glycerol.

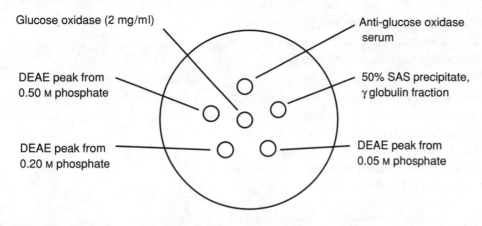

Glucose oxidase (2 mg/ml)

Anti-glucose oxidase serum

DEAE peak from 0.50 M phosphate

50% SAS precipitate, γ globulin fraction

DEAE peak from 0.20 M phosphate

DEAE peak from 0.05 M phosphate

FIGURE 4.2

Preparation of round gel plate. The distance between adjacent wells should be no more than 5–6 mm.

Questions

1. Do bands appear between the expected wells?

2. Can the relative molecular weights of glucose oxidase and antibody be determined by curvature of the bands?

Remember, small molecular weight proteins will diffuse more quickly through a matrix than large proteins.

Format 2: Preparation of microscope slide gel plate to detect IgG class antibody

DAY ONE

7. Pipette 3 ml agarose solution prepared in Step 1 onto each of two microscope slides placed on a flat bench. This amount of liquid is held on the plate by surface tension, but be careful not to release the agarose too quickly or it will run off the edges. Allow to set thoroughly, about 5 min.

An additional microscope plate may be prepared also, and its center trough filled with an anti-IgM serum, to verify the presence of IgM in any of the fractions.

8. Cut and remove the agarose from a number of 2 mm holes laterally on both long sides of the plate with a blunt-tipped 16-gauge needle by aspiration. Then cut a central trough with the double-edged razor blade knife (see Figure 4.3).

9. Pipette 2–3 μl DEAE fractions (Steps 6 and 7, Experiment 2,I,B) into successive wells on the plate. A micropipet with a 10–20 μl total capacity works best to avoid overfilling the wells. Next, fill the trough with 150–200 μl anti-goat (or sheep or rabbit) IgG and allow the solutions to diffuse overnight to develop the precipitin bands. During the incubation, place the plates in a humid atmosphere, for example, a Petri dish with moist filter paper on the bottom.

DAY TWO

10. Bands will appear opposite the wells containing IgG eluted from the DEAE column; thus, this technique can determine which fractions should be pooled for further purification.

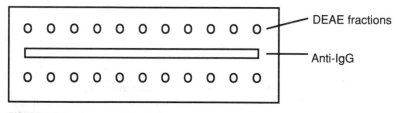

FIGURE 4.3

Preparation of microscope slide gel plate.

II. Immunoelectrophoresis

Immunoelectrophoresis (IEP) often is used instead of Ouchterlony double diffusion to obtain clearer precipitin patterns in complex antigen mixtures. The antigen sample first is electrophoresed through agarose gel and then is allowed to diffuse toward an antiserum to form precipitin bands (Figure 4.4). Because the sample is separated by electrophoresis before exposure to antibody, several antigens may be

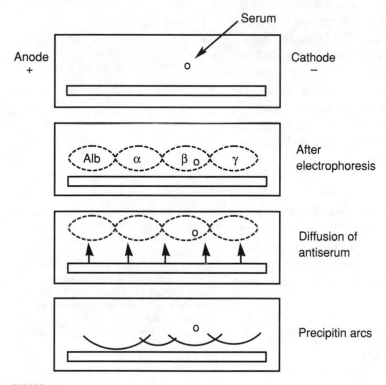

FIGURE 4.4

Immunoelectrophoresis.

identified if a polyspecific antiserum is used. Thus, immunoelectrophoresis often is used to make a tentative identification of an antigen in an unknown mixture or to follow the disappearance of contaminating antigens during a purification. Its main use in the clinical laboratory is to identify abnormal synthesis of immunoglobulins (myelomas and Bench–Jones proteins) and genetic protein variants with minor electrophoretic changes.

Electroendosmosis, heat, and pH shifts are phenomena that affect migration of sample molecules during electrophoresis. Many support matrixes absorb OH^- ions to their surfaces, resulting in a net increase in positive ions distant from the matrix. These positive ions migrate toward the negative pole with a solvent shell, resulting in a net solvent flow called *endosmosis*. Sample molecules migrating opposite these ions meet a resistance and are hindered in their travel. The larger the negative charge on the matrix, the greater the endosmotic effect. Cellulose, cellulose acetate, and agar gels may have strong electroendosmotic effects, but purified agarose has minimal surface charge and low endosmosis. Heat generated by a high ionic strength buffer also may affect sample migration. If the gel is cooled insufficiently during high voltage electrophoresis, the heat generated may melt the gel or denature the proteins. Finally, because the pH of the buffer may change due to the electrolysis of water, frequent buffer changes are necessary.

Experiment

In this experiment, the fractions obtained during the purification of anti-glucose oxidase IgG in Experiment 2 will be analyzed for purity by immunoelectrophoresis. This procedure views the anti-glucose oxidase samples as antigens, rather than antibodies. A polyspecific antiserum capable of reacting with all goat serum proteins will detect both contaminating proteins and the IgG fraction.

Materials

□ reagents and equipment used in Ouchterlony double diffusion

□ agarose, low electroendosmosis type (Sigma, BioRad)

□ anti-goat (or sheep or rabbit) whole serum

□ pure goat (or sheep or rabbit) IgG, 2 mg/ml

Barbitone is a Drug Enforcement Administration (DEA) controlled substance, and may be purchased only with proper license. Barbital buffer may be obtained from Beckman as Paragon B-2 buffer or from Gelman as High Resolution buffer without license. These buffers contain 12 gm sodium barbital and 4.40 gm barbital (must be dissolved in hot water) in 1 liter water. Mix the two together and adjust the pH to 8.6 with slow addition of 1 N NaOH to avoid precipitation of the barbital.

□ 0.05 M barbital buffer, pH 8.2–8.6

□ bromophenol blue, 0.5% solution in water

□ electrophoresis apparatus [e.g., Beckman Microzone (discontinued); Gelman Sepratek (#51156)]

Procedure

DAY ONE

1. Prepare 50 ml of 1.5–2% (w/v) agarose in barbital buffer by adding dry agarose to the buffer and heating just to boiling. (Be careful to heat the agarose solution slowly, or scorching and frothing will occur!)

2. Place two microscope slides on a level table top and quickly pipette 3 ml agarose onto each slide, spreading while releasing the agarose. The surface should be smooth; if not, try again. Allow to solidify for 5 min.

3. Remove two 2-mm wells with a blunt-tipped 16-guage needle in the plate, off center, by aspiration (Figure 4.5). Next, cut a center trough with razor blades, but do not remove the trough!

Commercial electrophoresis equipment is available, but is expensive for the occasional user. The Beckman and Gelman cells may be converted easily for IEP use by removing the membrane bridge and simply placing the slides across the buffer chambers. Filter paper wicks layed across the ends of the slides, dipping into the buffer, complete the electric circuit.

The slightly higher percentage of agarose (1.5–2%) compared with that used in Ouchterlony diffusion (1%) is used in IEP to produce a harder gel. Often the heat generated during electrophoresis softens lower percentage gels.

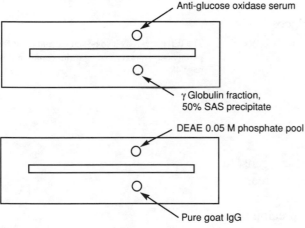

FIGURE 4.5

Preparing slide gels for immunoelectrophoresis.

4. Apply 2 µl of the various fractions to the wells (Figure 4.5). Wait a few minutes for the samples to absorb into the gel, and apply an additional 2 µl. Add a fraction of a microliter of 0.05% bromophenol blue as a marker to the well containing anti-glucose oxidase antiserum. The blue dye binds to albumin and indicates the migration rate of albumin toward the anode. Unbound bromophenol blue migrates faster than albumin.

5. Apply a current of 8 mA/slide for 30–60 min, or until the blue albumin dot nears the anode. The voltage should be 200–250 V.

6. Remove the troughs and add 100 µl anti- whole serum to each trough. The anti-goat whole serum will form precipitin bands with all serum proteins. The anti-glucose oxidase fractions will develop bands corresponding to the different proteins present. If a fraction is one pure protein, only one band will develop.

If the electrophoresis buffer compartments are larger than ~500 ml each, the polarity of each run may be changed 3–5 times before fresh buffer is required. Otherwise, empty both compartments into a common container between runs, and reuse 3–5 times before replacing buffer. Store all buffers at 4°C with 0.01% thimerosal as a bacteriostatic agent.

7. Place the plate in a Petri dish containing a moist piece of filter paper and allow diffusion at room temperature overnight to visualize precipitin bands.

DAY TWO

8. Identify any precipitin bands and compare placement of anti-glucose oxidase bands with the band seen with pure goat IgG. Store plates in refrigerator to preserve the bands.

The IEP plates may also be stained and dried for permanent storage, see margin comment on page 48.

III. Radial Immunodiffusion

Radial immunodiffusion (RID) is a quantitative assay for precipitable antigens. In this assay, the antibody is incorporated into a thin layer of agarose, whereas the protein antigen diffuses radially from a well. White rings are seen when the antigen concentration is optimal for precipitation; larger circles of precipitation indicate increased antigen concentration. This method is moderately sensitive, detecting 1–10 µg protein, and does not require pure antigen for concentration determination. However, it does take 24–48 hr to complete and only the presence, not the function, of the protein is assured. Commercial kits are available for many serum and clinically important proteins

Experiment

In this experiment, the concentration of an unknown sample of glucose oxidase will be determined by RID. Known concentrations of glucose oxidase will be provided to generate a standard curve. The concentration of unknown glucose oxidase samples then will be extrapolated from this curve.

Materials

- ☐ anti-glucose oxidase serum
- ☐ glucose oxidase standards, 5.0, 2.5, 1.2, and 0.62 mg/ml in PBS
- ☐ glucose oxidase unknowns, ranging from 0.5 to 5.0 mg/ml
- ☐ agar or agarose
- ☐ buffer composed of 0.15 M NaCl, 0.01 M Tris, pH 7.5–8.0, 0.005 M EDTA, 0.02% NaN_3
- ☐ 100-mm Petri dishes
- ☐ microscope slides
- ☐ 60°C water bath

Procedure

DAY ONE

1. Prepare 50 ml 1% (w/v) agarose in the buffer, slowly heating to a gentle boil to dissolve. Place dissolved agarose in a 60°C water bath and allow to equilibrate.

    CAUTION! Watch out for sudden frothing when near boiling.

2. Place a clean microscope slide on a level bench top.

3. Place an empty 13 × 150-mm test tube in the 60°C water bath and add 0.1–0.3 ml of anti-glucose oxidase (see margin note). Allow a few minutes

for the antiserum to equilibrate to 60°C, then add 3 ml warm agarose and mix quickly by inverting once or twice, using parafilm to cover the tube. Immediately place the tube in 60°C water bath to prevent gelling.

4. Use a disposable plastic or pasteur pipet to transfer the entire agarose–antiserum mixture quickly but smoothly onto the microscope plate. Be sure to "push" any bubbles to the edges. Work quickly! Allow to solidify for 5 min.

5. Remove agarose from 6 wells, 2 mm in diameter by aspiration in the agarose-coated plate with a blunt 16-gauge needle (see Figure 4.6).

6. Apply 2 μl of each of 4 standard solutions to the first 4 wells and 2 μl of the unknown to the 5th and 6th wells. Use a Hamilton syringe or a 10-μl micropipet with a narrow tip.

7. Place the plate gently into a Petri dish containing moist filter paper. Replace lid and allow to incubate at room temperature 24–48 hr to develop precipitin rings.

DAY TWO

8. Measure the ring diameter in millimeters. Plot the square of the diameter against the concentration of the standards. Determine the concentration of the unknown by extrapolation from the standard curve.

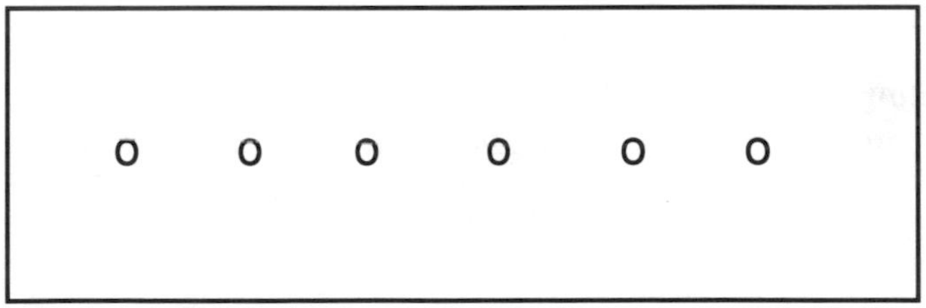

Antibodies can maintain their native structure up to approximately 65°C for short periods of time. Thus, it is important to maintain an accurate 60°C to avoid antibody denaturation and loss of function.

Instructor's Note : The correct amount of anti-glucose oxidase serum to use will vary with different antisera. Thus, it is prudent to predetermine the optimal volume that gives the largest circles with the glucose oxidase standards. Alternatively, if enough anti-glucose oxidase is available, the student may determine the optimal volume by making several plates.

FIGURE 4.6

Pattern used to punch wells in agarose-coated plate.

REFERENCES

Clausen, J. (1977). "Immunochemical Techniques for the Identification and Estimation of Macromolecules." North-Holland, Amsterdam.

Ouchterlony, O., and Nilsson, L.-A. (1986). Immunodiffusion and immunoelectrophoresis. *In* "Handbook of Experimental Immunology (D. M.Weir, L. A. Herzenberg, and C. Blackwell, eds.), Vol. 1, pp. 32.1–32.50. Blackwell, Oxford.

Affinity Chromatography of Antibodies

In affinity chromatography, a specific molecule is purified away from others by binding to an insolubilized, immobilized ligand. For the purification of antibodies, the ligand is the antigen covalently linked to an insoluble support. This discussion will consider supports and chemistries for ligand attachment, elution conditions, and, finally, other types of affinity procedures. The experimental section shows how to prepare and use an affinity support to purify anti-glucose oxidase antibody.

Insoluble Supports and Ligand Attachment Reactions

Polysaccharide Supports

The most common insoluble support for affinity chromatography is agarose gel, termed Sepharose by its manufacturer, Pharmacia. Agarose is an amorphous polysaccharide consisting of neutral galactose residues in helical bundles. Cellulose in the form of paper or fibers also may be used for specific applications.

Whether agarose or cellulose is used, the polysaccharide first must be activated so it can bind the ligand. The most common activating agent for agarose is cyanogen bromide (CNBr), which forms a covalent isourea linkage with a ligand that contains an amino group (Axen *et al.*, 1967; Parikh *et al.*, 1974; Scouten, 1987). This linkage is somewhat unstable for long periods of time, either in the presence of nucleophiles (e.g., azide and Tris buffers) or at extreme pHs. Carbonyldiimidazole and bis-oxiranes are also useful activating agents, but the activation procedures for these agents are more complex and are used only if necessary. Activated resins are available commercially (BioRad, Pharmacia, Pierce, Sigma) but may be produced easily in the laboratory at a considerable savings, often with increased binding capacity.

$$\begin{array}{c} NH \\ \parallel \\ -O-C-NH-R \end{array}$$

Isourea linkage. See Appendix A for details on this and other linkage chemistries for affinity chromatography.

Polyacrylamide Support

Another popular support resin is polyacrylamide, sold as BioGel-P (BioRad). Polyacrylamide may be activated with a number of agents, the most common of which is gluteraldehyde, which activates the resin to bind amino-containing ligands. The resultant Schiff base is chemically very stable and is used often if CNBr–agarose leaches excessive ligand. If the ligand does not contain an amino group, alternative chemistries may be used for both agarose and polyacrylamide that allow carboxyl, sulfhydryl, and aldehyde groups on ligands to be attached (Table 5.1) (Inman and Dintzis, 1969; Bethell *et al.*, 1979).

—CH$_2$—NH—R
Reduced Schiff base

Effective Binding of Ligand to Support

The chemistries listed in Table 5.1 provide wide latitude in the possible linkages between the ligand and the support. Consequently, the optimal chemistry for ligand binding should be considered when designing an affinity support. For example, the ε-amino of lysine is the predominant group that binds protein antigens to a CNBr-activated support. These amino groups are spread randomly throughout a protein, resulting in a bound protein with many orientations on the support. Thus, effective binding of antibody to such an antigen–support complex will depend on whether the epitopes are oriented correctly to be recognized by the

The correct support and activation procedure to use for a particular affinity problem cannot be determined by theory alone. It is often necessary to try a procedure and determine its effectiveness, and then try another. For instance, one procedure may bind more antigen to a resin initially than another procedure, but it may result in leaching of the ligand during elution or it may cause the ligand to be hindered sterically and bind antibody poorly.

TABLE 5-1

Affinity Chromatography Chemistries

Support	Activating agent	Ligand reactive group
Agarose	CNBr	amino
	CNBr + diamine	carboxyl, using CDI[a]
	carbonyldiimidazole	amino
	bis-oxirane	amino, hydroxyl
	periodate	amino
Polyacrylamide	gluteraldehyde	amino
	hydroxide (OH$^-$)	amino, using CDI
	ethylenediamine	carboxyl, using CDI
	hydrazine	aldehyde

[a] CDI, Carbodiimide; a water soluble version is 1-ethyl-3-(3-dimethylaminopropyl) carbodiimide hydrochloride.

antibody. This may not be a problem with polyclonal antibodies, which have many binding specificities, but monoclonal antibodies may be more sensitive to antigen orientation on the support. In addition, certain amino acids in proteins are critical for antibody binding, so appropriate chemistries should be chosen to avoid masking these amino acids.

Elution Conditions for Affinity Chromatography

Affinity Chromatography of Antibodies

During affinity column chromatographic purification of antibodies, the impure antibody preparation is allowed to pass through a column of the antigen-modified support. The antibodies specific for the antigen bind to the column, and impurities are washed from the column with large amounts of buffer. The specific antibodies then are released from the column by the addition of a buffer that disrupts the antigen–antibody bond. The trick in this procedure is to use the mildest condition that effectively releases the antibody. Normally, denaturing conditions are necessary to break the ionic, hydrophobic, and hydrogen bonds that hold the antigen and antibody together. Thus, antibody recovery from denaturing conditions varies, depending on the types and number of bonds holding antibody to antigen, the subclass of antibody, and the type of denaturant. The most common denaturing condition is low pH, 2.1–3.0, after which the antibody is brought immediately to pH 7 to minimize exposure to acid conditions. Other agents used to release antibodies include the chaotropic salts NaSCN and KBr; the organic solvents ethanol, acetonitrile and dioxane, and detergents such as SDS. All eluting conditions result in some loss of antibody function, either in the antigen binding sites or in the "effector" regions distant from the binding sites. Only empirical evidence can determine which elution condition is best for a specific antibody preparation. Unfortunately, very high affinity antibodies, which may be the most valuable for immunoassays, may be difficult to elute from an affinity column. In addition, any antibody remaining on the affinity column will lower the capacity of the column for subsequent purifications.

Small organic molecules also may be bound to a support and used in affinity purification of anti-hapten antibodies. Elution of anti-hapten antibodies usually is

A chaotropic compound is one that causes chaos in the system studied. In immunoaffinity techniques, the chaotrope is used to break the ligand–antibody interaction.

61

accomplished by competing off the antibodies with a close *analog* of the hapten. For example, trinitrophenol analog may be used to dislodge an anti-dinitrophenol antibody. The analog is used in high concentrations, 0.1–0.5 M, and the released antibody carries the analog in its binding site. The analog then is removed by extensive dialysis, gel filtration, or by passage of the analog–antibody through an ion-exchange column (charged analogs). Of course, denaturing conditions also may be used to dislodge the analog from the antibody.

If the original hapten were used to compete the antibody off the affinity resin, the hapten would be extremely difficult to remove from the eluted hapten–antibody complex without denaturation of the antibody.

Immunoaffinity Purification of Antigens

Antibodies bound to a support have been used increasingly to purify antigens from complex mixtures. The choices of antibody and elution conditions are of primary importance in this technique to preserve the structure and function of the antigen.

Polyclonal or monoclonal antibodies may be used on affinity supports. A polyclonal offers a broad specificity for the antigen and a range of binding affinities, whereas a single monoclonal offers a single binding specificity and a single binding affinity. Because of the heterogeneity of antigen binding by polyclonals, complete release of the antigen may require several different, and perhaps harsh, elution conditions. In contrast, monoclonal antibodies bind the antigen at only one epitope, and often release the antigen with a very specific elution condition that may be gentler than that needed with polyclonals. However, polyclonals are often easier to obtain than monoclonals, and may be quite satisfactory for some studies.

The conditions needed to elute an antigen from an antibody are not necessarily reflected in the affinity of the antibody for antigen; high affinity antibodies may release their antigens as easily as low affinity antibodies. Since all antibodies bind antigen with ionic, hydrophobic, and hydrogen bonding interactions, the susceptibility of these bonds to elution conditions is independent of affinity. In general, high affinity antibodies are desirable to bind all antigen molecules from an impure mixture effectively. Thus, high affinity monoclonal antibodies may be the ideal reagents with which to purify antigens, but only empirical results will show which antibodies, linkage chemistries, and elution conditions will be most effective for any particular application.

Other Antibody Affinity Purification Techniques

At times, scientists wish to purify all immunoglobulins of a certain class from a mixture instead of only one specific antibody. Protein A from *Staphylococcus aureus* and Protein G from group G *Streptococcus* are cell-surface proteins that bind the Fc portion of antibody molecules (Lindmark *et al.*, 1983; Bjorck and Kronvall, 1984; Akerstrom *et al.*, 1985). Thus, proteins A and G bound to supports are used to affinity purify a class of immunoglobulins. Although there are some species and subclass limitations, proteins A and G often are used in purifying IgG from monoclonal antibody sources and in situations in which no effective purification procedures have succeeded. Low pH (3–4) is the typical elution condition for these proteins.

Antibodies with specificity for classes and subclasses of immunoglobulins also have been used to purify antibody. Like proteins A and G, the use of anti-immunoglobulins allow the purification of one class of antibody, whereas elution conditions require the same disrupting agents used in immunoaffinity chromatography.

Experiment

In this experiment, an affinity support will be made by attaching glucose oxidase to CNBr-activated agarose. Anti-glucose oxidase antibody then will be purified with this affinity support. In subsequent experiments, the purified antibody will be labeled (Experiment 6) and used in immunoblotting and enzyme immunoassay (Experiments 7 and 10).

Materials

□ anti-glucose oxidase IgG obtained from DEAE (Step 9, Experiment 2)

□ CNBr-activated gel (Method A, Appendix A)

□ glucose oxidase (Sigma #G 7016)

□ aminoethanol

□ 0.1 M sodium carbonate, pH 9

□ 1 M NaCl, 0.01 M potassium phosphate, pH 7.4

Protein A and G Bind IgG Subclasses Differently[a]

Source	Subclass	Protein A	Protein G
bird	all	–	+
bovine	IgG1	–	++
bovine	IgG2	++	++
guinea pig	IgG1,2	++	+
goat	IgG1,2	+	++
human	IgG1,2,4	++	++
human	IgG3	+	++
human	IgM	(+)	
human	IgA2	(+)	
human	IgA1	–	
mouse	IgG1	+	++
mouse	IgG2a,b,3	++	++
pig	IgG1,2	++	++
pig	IgM	+	
rabbit	IgG	++	++
rat	IgG1	+	+
rat	IgG2a,b	–	++
rat	IgG2c	++	++
sheep	IgG1	–	++
sheep	IgG2	++	++

[a]++, Strong; +, Weak; – No binding.

To weigh CNBr, tare an empty screw-capped wide-mouth bottle. Then, in the fume hood, transfer the CNBr to the bottle and reweigh. The difference is the weight of CNBr. Finally, add enough acetonitrile to dissolve the CNBr. The mixture will become cold; warming may be necessary for complete dissolution.

- ☐ 1 M NaCl, 0.01 M sodium acetate, pH 4.5
- ☐ 0.2 M glycine–HCl, pH 2.5
- ☐ 0.2 M Tris–HCl, pH 8.0
- ☐ PBS (Appendix B)
- ☐ 15-ml screw-capped plastic conical centrifuge tube
- ☐ 10-ml plastic syringe barrel

I. Preparation of Affinity Resin

Procedure

DAY ONE

ACTIVATION OF RESIN AND ADDITION OF GLUCOSE OXIDASE

1. Activate Sepharose with CNBr (see Method A, Appendix A). The activation will be done by the instructor to avoid exposure of the students to toxic CNBr. After activation, each student will receive approximately 5 ml activated gel as a moist "cake." Keep on ice until needed.

2. Dissolve 25 mg glucose oxidase in 5 ml 0.10 M sodium carbonate, pH 9.0. Carefully transfer 0.20 ml into a test tube and add 1.80 ml 0.1 M sodium carbonate, pH 9.0. Seal and save at 4°C for later use (Step 7). Use remaining glucose oxidase solution in Step 3.

   The final protein bound to the gel should be between 0.1 and 10 mg/ml gel. Generally, 2–5 mg/ml gel is optimal to avoid steric hindrance.

3. Add approximately 4 ml activated Sepharose to 4 ml glucose oxidase solution in a 15-ml plastic conical centrifuge tube. Gently agitate on a shaker overnight, either at 4°C or at room temperature.

   Shaking the support at 4°C is safest for labile proteins. Stirring the agarose support with a magnetic stir bar should be avoided to minimize fragmentation of the agarose beads.

DAY TWO

POURING AND WASHING COLUMN

4. The next morning, add 0.10 ml aminoethanol to the mixture and continue shaking for an additional 2 hr or longer. The aminoethanol binds any unreacted sites on the support and donates a neutral OH group.

5. Pour the slurry into a vertically mounted 10-ml plastic syringe barrel with glass wool at the bottom. Save the material (that contains unbound glucose oxidase) that drips out of the bottom of the syringe as the column packs, and add an additional 4.0 ml 0.10 M sodium carbonate, pH 9.0 to wash the column. Combine both washes to quantitate the amount of unbound glucose oxidase (see Step 7).

6. Wash the column successively with 10 ml 1.0 M NaCl, 0.01 M potassium phosphate, pH 7.4; 10 ml 1.0 M NaCl, 0.01 M sodium acetate, pH 4.5; 20 ml PBS. (Discard all washes.)

The 1 M NaCl and low pH acetate will remove noncovalently bound glucose oxidase molecules. The hydrogen and ionic bonding that may be holding proteins to the agarose noncovalently is minimized with high salt and low pH conditions.

7. Determine the amount of glucose oxidase bound to your column by absorption spectrophotometry. First, measure the absorbance at 280 nm of the glucose oxidase dilution prepared in Step 2. Using this absorbance, calculate the milligrams of glucose oxidase added to the support. Second, measure the absorbance at 280 nm of the washes containing the unbound material obtained in Step 5. Use this absorbance to calculate the milligrams of glucose oxidase not bound to the support. For both calculations, use an extinction coefficient of 1.68 for 1 mg/ml glucose oxidase. Third, subtract the milligrams of unbound glucose oxidase from the added glucose oxidase. The difference is the glucose oxidase bound to the column, which should be at least 1–2 mg glucose oxidase bound per ml packed gel.

8. Drain the column until the level of PBS buffer is just below the top of the column. The column is now ready to receive the antibody sample. If the column is not used immediately, store at 4°C before draining.

II. Affinity Chromatography

DAY ONE

LOADING AND ELUTION OF THE AFFINITY COLUMN

9. Measure the total volume of anti-glucose oxidase IgG obtained from the DEAE pool; save 0.2–0.5 ml for calculating final yield if not already done. Apply the DEAE-purified anti-glucose oxidase to the affinity column, saving all elutions. After the antibody has gone through the column once, reapply the antibody to insure efficient binding.

Remember, the glucose oxidase is on a solid phase and the antibody must have time to diffuse throughout the resin to bind to the antigen.

10. After application of the antibody, wash the column with 20 ml 1 M NaCl, 0.01 M potassium phosphate, pH 7.4, followed by 20 ml 1 M NaCl, 0.01 M sodium acetate, pH 4.5. Drain the last wash to the surface of the support.

11. Prepare 15 test tubes (13 × 150 mm), each containing 1 ml 0.2 M Tris, pH 8.0. Apply 1 ml 0.2 M glycine, pH 2.5, to the top of the column. Allow this solution to soak into the column while collecting the 1 ml eluted directly into one of the Tris-filled tubes. Continue the addition and collection of 14 more 1-ml fractions of the 0.2 M glycine. Wait about 2 min between fractions to allow time for antibody desorption from the gel. Read the A_{280} for each tube. Combine the fractions that contain the majority of the eluted antibody. If one or two tubes have especially high concentrations, 1 mg/ml or greater, dialyze separately and use for peroxidase and biotin conjugation (Experiment 6).

12. Dialyze all antibody containing fractions against several changes of 0.15 M NaCl (8.5 gm/liter) at 4°C.

13. Calculate the milligrams of anti-glucose oxidase purified from the affinity column, using an absorbance at 280 nm of 1.35 for antibody. Next, determine the percentage yield of this affinity pure anti-glucose oxidase from (1) the original antiserum (Step 1, Experiment 2,I,A) and (2) the DEAE IgG pool (Step 9, Experiment 2,I,B).

14. Store at least 1 ml anti-glucose oxidase frozen for ELISA (Experiment 10) and save the rest to be labeled with peroxidase or biotin (Experiment 6).

Instead of a DEAE-purified sample, many researchers apply raw antisera or ascites directly to the affinity column. This is possible because of the extreme purifications obtained with affinity methods, often 10,000 fold. If crude starting preparations are used, the washing of the column must be thorough to insure complete removal of contaminating proteins.

Questions

What is the percentage of glucose oxidase applied to the column that became attached to the Sepharose in Step 7?

Was the glucose oxidase affinity column yellow? What chemical produces the yellow color? Did the yellow color elute from the affinity column during the acid elution of Step 11? Why? Finally, did the yellow color remain in the bag following dialysis in Step 12? Why?

REFERENCES

Akerstrom, B., Brodin, T., Reis, K., and Bjorck, L. (1985). Protein G: A powerful tool for binding and detection of monoclonal and polyclonal antibodies. *J. Immunol.* **135**, 2589–2592.

Axen, R., Porath, J., and Ernback, S. (1967). Chemical coupling of peptides and proteins to polysaccharides by means of cyanogen halides. *Nature (London)* **214**, 1302–1304.

Bethell, G. S., Ayers, J. S., Hancock, W. S., and Hearn, M. T. (1979). A novel method of activation of cross-linked agaroses with 1,1′-carbonyldiimidazole which gives a matrix for affinity chromatography devoid of additional charged groups. *J. Biol. Chem.* **254**, 2572–2574.

Bjorck, L. and Kronvall, G. (1984). Purification and some properties of streptococcal protein G, a novel IgG-binding reagent. *J. Immunol.* **133**, 969–974.

Inman, J. K. and Dintzis, H. M. (1969). The derivatization of cross-linked polyacrylamide beads. Controlled introduction of functional groups for preparation of special purpose, biochemical adsorbents. *Biochemistry* **8**, 4074.

Lindmark, R., Thoren-Tolling, K., and Sjoquist, J. (1983). Binding of immunoglobulins to protein A and immunoglobulin levels in mammalian sera. *J. Immunol. Methods* **62**, 1–13.

Parikh, I., March, S., and Cuatrecasas, P. (1974). Topics in the methodology of substitution reactions with agarose. *Meth. Enzymol.* **34**, 77–102.

Scouten, W. H. (1987). A survey of enzyme coupling techniques. In "Immobilization Techniques for Enzymes" (Klaus Mosbach, ed.), pp. 31–64. Academic Press, New York.

Labeling Antibodies

Antibodies modified with a *label* often are used to detect antigens in a variety of immunochemical techniques. The labeled antibody binds to the antigen and then is detected by using the label as a signal. The most common labels are enzymes and radioactivity, but fluorophores, colloidal gold, and heavy metals are used also. The choice of label depends on the end use: enzyme and radioactive labels are very effective in blot and ELISA techniques, while fluorescent and metal labels are particularly useful in flow cytometry and immunocytochemistry. The discussion section for this experiment focuses on both direct and indirect enzyme labels, whereas the experimental section provides protocols for proxidase, alkaline phosphatase, and biotin. Investigators commonly link these labels to primary antibodies for use in blot and ELISA techniques. The low backgrounds and reduced number of incubation steps obtained when using labeled primary antibody are often worth the extra effort of the labeling procedure. However, investigators do not normally label primary antibodies with fluorescent or metal labels for use in FACS and immunocytochemistry work. The monoclonal antibodies extensively used in these techniques are effectively detected by commercially available fluorescent- or metal-labeled secondary antibodies. Protocols for labeling with radioactive iodine are given in Appendix G.

Enzyme Labels

The criteria for an ideal enzyme label include high specific activity, low cost, effectiveness of coupling, absence from biological samples, stability in storage, and ease of assay. The most widely used enzymes are horseradish peroxidase (HRP), alkaline phosphatase (AP), and β-galactosidase. The choice of which enzyme to use is often a personal preference, but some considerations include that interfering peroxidases and phosphatases occur in some biological samples, that certain substrates may be toxic or unstable, and that some enzymes produce a better linear response. Horseradish peroxidase will be used in this experiment,

TABLE 6-1

Enzymes Used as Labels with Antibodies[a]

Enzyme	Linkage chemistry	Substrates	Comments	Reference
Peroxidase	glutaraldehyde; periodate oxidation	OPD, ATBS (soluble) DAB, CN (insoluble)	Peroxidase activities in leukocytes; substrates toxic	Avarmeas *et al.* (1979) Nakane (1979)
Alkaline phosphatase	glutaraldehyde	NPP, MUP (soluble) BCIP, NBT (insoluble)	Phosphatase activities in some tissues	Avrameas (1969) Engvall and Perlman (1971)
β-Galactosidase	glutaraldehyde; MBS	ONPG (soluble) BCIG (insoluble)	No enzyme in eukaryotic tissues; low background in histochemistry	O'Sullivan *et al.* (1979) O'Sullivan and Marks (1981)

[a]Abbreviations: ATBS, 2,2′-azinodi-(3-ethylbenzothiazoline-6-sulfonic acid); BCIG, 5-bromo-4-chloro-3-indolyl—D-galactopyranoside; BCIP, 5-bromo-4-chloro-3-indolyl phosphate; CN, 4-chloronaphthol; DAB, 3,3′-diaminobenzidine; MBS, *m*-maleimidobenzoyl-*N*-hydroxysuccinimide ester; MUP, 4-methyl umbelliferyl phosphate (fluorogenic); NBT, nitro blue tetrazolium; NPP, *p*-nitrophenyl phosphate; ONPG, *o*-nitrophenyl—D-galactoside; OPD, *o*-phenylene-diamine.

both because it has an extremely high turnover number and because it may be coupled to many different antibodies consistently. Alkaline phosphatase may be the enzyme of choice when extreme sensitivity is needed, since fluorescent and chemiluminescent substrates offer a 10-fold increase in sensitivity over chromogenic substrates. Alkaline phosphatase and β-galactosidase also generate product in amounts that correlate closely to the amount of enzyme present, making them useful for quantitation on blot assays.

Labeling Chemistries

Enzymes may be attached to antibodies by direct or indirect methods. The *direct methods* link enzyme to antibody covalently whereas the *indirect methods* use an intermediate molecule to link the enzyme noncovalently. Since both methods offer advantages, examples of each will be used in our experiment.

Direct Methods

Direct coupling of enzymes to antibodies must preserve the activity of both the enzyme and the antibody. Although there is no single chemistry that is equally successful for all enzyme–antibody systems, glutaraldehyde has been reasonably successful for most enzymes (see Figure 6.2). This reagent links amino groups on an enzyme to amino groups on an antibody. Because some amino groups may be in or near the antibody binding site, the antigen-binding ability of the antibody may be reduced when an enzyme is linked to these amino groups. If this occurs, chemistries may be used that link the enzyme to either the carbohydrate or the sulfhydryl groups on the antibody, distant from the antigen-binding site. Most labeling chemistries form large-molecular-weight heterogenous antibody–enzyme conjugates, with an average of less than one enzyme coupled per antibody. Despite the large size and the heterogeneity of these conjugates, they work remarkably well in most immunochemical assays.

Direct labeling offers two advantages: background signal is low because the label is directly attached to the specific antibody, and the number of reagents in the assay is held to a minimum. However, there are also two disadvantages. First, a purified polyclonal or monoclonal antibody is required for labeling and, second, each different antibody must be labeled. For a busy laboratory, this results in purifying and labeling many antibodies, a somewhat onerous task.

Indirect Methods: Protein A and Biotin–Streptavidin

Indirect methods do not link an enzyme directly to an antibody. Instead, they use an enzyme-labeled (secondary) molecule that binds to the (primary) antibody in a second step of the assay. Indirect methods often result in the attachment of several enzyme molecules to each primary antibody molecule, offering an amplification over direct methods (Figure 6.1). Two of the most popular secondary molecules are streptavidin and protein A (or protein G).

Streptavidin is an effective secondary molecule when used with the vitamin *biotin*. Biotin is a low molecular weight molecule with a strong noncovalent affinity ($K_a \sim 10^{15}$ M^{-1}) for the protein streptavidin, the extracellular product of *Streptomyces avidinii*. Because of this unusually high affinity, the biotin—streptavidin system has found wide use in the immunoassay field (Wilchek and Bayer, 1988; Green, 1990). In use, a primary antibody is labeled with biotin and allowed to form the specific antibody complex. An enzyme–streptavidin conjugate (available commercially) then is used as the secondary label to bind the biotin-labeled antibody (Figure 6.1B). Because the biotin–antibody complex often binds more than one enzyme–streptavidin conjugate, the final number of enzyme molecules associated with the antigen–antibody complex is often greater than with

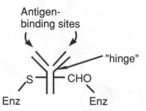

Specific chemistries may link enzyme (Enz) to either sulfhydryl (S) or carbohydrate (CHO) groups near the hinge region of the antibody.

Avidin from egg white also binds biotin strongly and is effective as a secondary molecule. However, streptavidin is often preferred over avidin because streptavidin is negatively charged and contains no carbohydrate. Consequently, streptavidin exhibits less nonspecific binding with antigen samples that contain either endogenous chromatin, heparin, or acidic proteins (all of which are negatively charged) or lectins (proteins that bind carbohydrates).

Comparison of Avidin and Streptavidin

Protein	pI	Molecular weight	Number of subunits	Carbohydrate
Avidin	10	68,000	4	Yes
Streptavidin	5–6	60,000	4	No

Source: Green (1990).

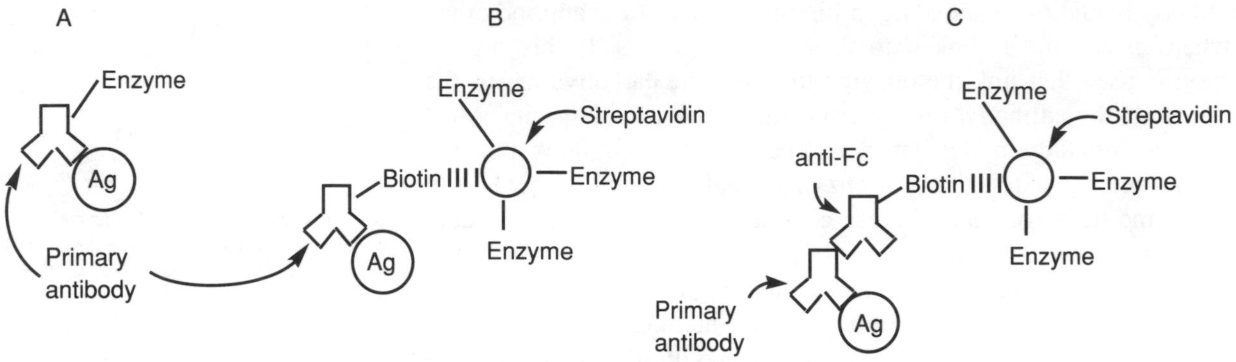

A   B   C

FIGURE 6.1

Amplification of enzyme label with biotin–streptavidin. (A) Direct labeling using enzyme–labeled antibody. (B) Indirect labeling using biotin–streptavidin. (C) Indirect labeling using biotin–anti-Fc intermediate.

a directly labeled antibody (Figure 6.1A). Thus, the biotin–streptavidin system often results in an amplification of final signal over that seen with directly labeled antibodies.

If it is difficult to label the primary antibody with biotin directly then an intermediate biotin-labeled anti-Fc may be employed. This conjugate specifically binds to the Fc regions of the primary antibody and serves to incorporate biotin for subsequent streptavidin binding (Figure 6.1C). The two advantages to this reagent are that no primary antibody needs to be purified (antiserum is often sufficient) and many different primary antibodies may be detected with only one biotin-labeled anti-Fc.

An alternative indirect method uses protein A, a bacterial protein found on the surface of certain *Streptococcus* strains. It binds avidly to the Fc portion of IgGs from many species (see Experiment 5). When conjugated with an enzyme, it may be used as the indirect enzyme label to bind the primary antibody. This method does not demand purification of the primary antibody, and requires only one enzyme–protein A reagent to detect many different primary antibodies.

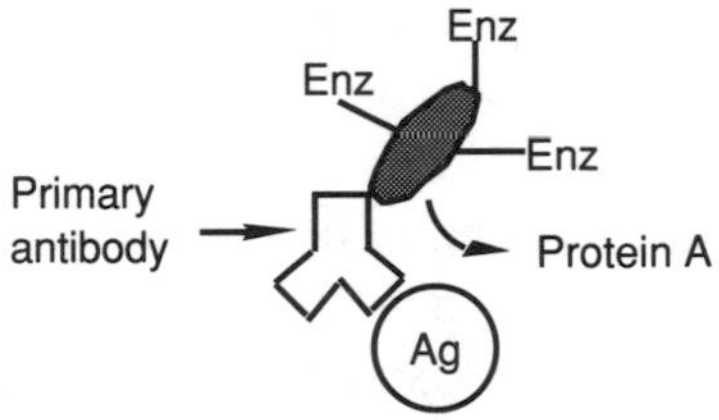

Indirect labeling with protein A intermediate.

Experiment

In this experiment, anti-glucose oxidase will be labeled with HRP, and biotin for use in enzyme-linked immunosorbent assay (Experiment 10) and blotting techniques (Experiment 7). The two different labels will allow comparison of the sensitivity of direct (HRP) and indirect (biotin) labels. A protocol for coupling the enzyme alkaline phosphatase is given immediately after the HRP procedure.

Coupling Peroxidase by Periodate Oxidation

HRP usually is coupled to antibody by the cross-linking agent glutaraldehyde or by periodate oxidation and subsequent Schiff base formation (Figures 6.2 and 6.3). In this experiment, the periodate method will be used since it produces HRP–antibody conjugates that usually require no postlabeling purification. Although conjugation of HRP to affinity-purified antibody is preferable, conjugation to a DEAE-purified IgG portion of antiserum may be satisfactory.

Enzyme–antibody conjugates occasionally produce either low sensitivity or high background in immunoassays. This may be caused by a fraction of high molecular weight material in the conjugate, which often is removed by gel filtration. Some procedures mask amino groups on the HRP with dinitrophenol to minimize inter-HRP cross-linking by glutaraldehyde. Such cross-linking might produce troublesome high molecular weight conjugates.

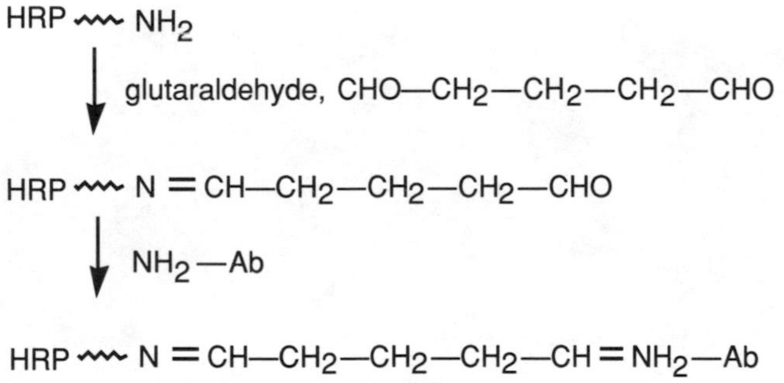

HRP $\sim\!\!\sim$ NH$_2$

$\downarrow$ glutaraldehyde, CHO—CH$_2$—CH$_2$—CH$_2$—CHO

HRP $\sim\!\!\sim$ N $=$ CH—CH$_2$—CH$_2$—CH$_2$—CHO

$\downarrow$ NH$_2$—Ab

HRP $\sim\!\!\sim$ N $=$ CH—CH$_2$—CH$_2$—CH$_2$—CH $=$ NH$_2$—Ab

FIGURE 6.2

Glutaraldehyde coupling of HRP to immunoglobulin.

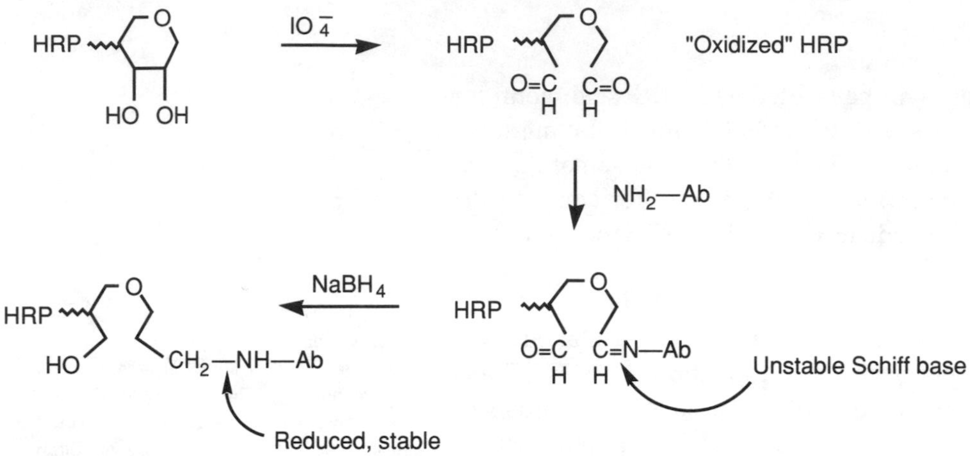

FIGURE 6.3

Periodate coupling of HRP to immunoglobulin.

Materials

- ☐ affinity-purified anti-glucose oxidase antibody (Step 6, Experiment 5,II)
- ☐ periodate-treated peroxidase (see Step 9)
  - horseradish peroxidase (Sigma #P6782)
  - sodium periodate ($NaIO_4$)
  - 1 mM sodium acetate, pH 4.4
  - dialysis tubing
- ☐ 1 M potassium carbonate, pH 9.5
- ☐ PBS (Appendix B)
- ☐ sodium borohydride ($NaBH_4$)
- ☐ 100% SAS
- ☐ Sephadex G-50 or dialysis tubing (see Step 7)

I. Peroxidase Labeling of Antibody

Procedure

This procedure is a modification of that of Voller *et al.* (1980).

DAY ONE

1. To the antibody solution (0.1–10 mg/ml in 0.15 M NaCl), add 1 M potassium carbonate, pH 9.5, to a final concentration of 0.01 M carbonate.

2. Add 0.5 mg periodate-treated HRP (about 4 mg/ml in 0.001 M acetate, pH 4.4) for every 1.0 mg antibody. The instructor will provide the oxidized HRP, but the procedure is given in Step 9. The pH of the final HRP–antibody mixture should be near 8.5–9.5; check by spotting 5–10 μl onto universal pH paper.

3. Incubate 1.5–2 hr at room temperature.

4. Add NaBH$_4$ to a final concentration of 0.2 mg/ml. To do this, add 0.1 ml 2.2 mg/ml NaBH$_4$ in water to every 1.0 ml of the antibody–HRP mixture. Swirl gently. Incubate at room temperature for 30 min.

5. Dialyze against PBS (or proceed directly to Step 6).

DAY TWO

6. Remove unconjugated HRP by precipitation of the HRP–antibody with 50% SAS. To save time, prepare a 10-ml Sephadex G-50 column during the SAS precipitation (see steps 7a–f). Add an equal volume of 100% SAS to the HRP–antibody mixture from Step 5. Pellet the HRP–antibody conjugate by centrifugation at 3000–5000 *g*. (Unconjugated HRP is discarded in the supernatant.) Wash the pellet once with 50% SAS and dissolve the final pellet in 0.5 ml PBS.

7. Remove excess ammonium sulfate from the dissolved HRP–antibody complex by dialyzing against PBS or by gel filtering through a Sephadex G-50 column (see a–f).

a. Pour approximately one heaping teaspoon (no more!) dry Sephadex G-50 into about 200 ml PBS. Stir to suspend and allow to swell for at least 30 min at room temperature.

b. Pour a 10-ml Sephadex G-50 column in a 10-ml glass pipet fitted with a small piece of tubing, and clamp to stop the flow. Wash the column with 10–15 ml PBS. Save the remaining G-50 in the refrigerator.

c. Drain all buffer to a level just at the top of the column.

d. Apply up to 1.0 ml HRP–antibody mixture; allow to drain into the column. If less than 1 ml mixture was added, apply enough PBS to total 1 ml. Discard all effluent.

e. Gently add two separate 0.5-ml aliquots PBS. Allow each aliquot to drain into the column before the next addition. Finally, add 1 ml PBS and drain into column. A total of 2 ml PBS have now been added. Discard all effluent.

f. Apply an additional 2 ml PBS. Immediately start collecting the effluent in a new tube, until the 2 ml have drained into the column. The 2 ml effluent contains the HRP–antibody complex.

8. Store the HRP–Ab at 4°C for short term storage.

9. Peroxidase oxidation procedure

a. To 4 mg peroxidase in 1 ml distilled water, add 0.2 ml freshly prepared 0.1 M NaIO$_4$ (21 mg/ml) and stir gently for 20 min. On addition of the periodate, the solution should change color from gold to green; if it does not do so, new NaIO$_4$ is required.

b. Dialyze the mixture against 1 mM sodium acetate buffer, pH 4.4, overnight at 4°C.

c. Use to conjugate to antibody within 1 day of preparation.

CAUTION! Since HRP is inhibited by low concentrations of azide, sodium azide should never be used to preserve any HRP conjugates. Store the conjugates long term at –20°C in 50% glycerol, at –70°C with BSA as carrier, or at 4°C after filter sterilization.

Optional Protocol

Coupling Alkaline Phosphatase
This procedure is adapted from O'Sullivan and Marks (1981).

1. To 1 mg antibody (0.5–2 mg/ml) in PBS, add 3 mg alkaline phosphatase.

2. Add glutaraldehyde to 0.20% with gentle vortexing.

3. Incubate 2 hr at room temperature.

4. Desalt by chromatography on Sephadex G-25 or dialysis against TBS buffer (Appendix B) containing 1 mM $MgCl_2$. Add BSA to 0.2% to the conjugate to increase stability. Store at 4°C after sterile filtration or addition of sodium azide to 0.02%.

Coupling Biotin Using a Succinimidyl Ester Derivative, NHS–Biotin

In this protocol, biotin will be coupled to random amino groups on antibody with a succinimidyl ester (NHS) biotin derivative (Figure 6.4). At low biotin–antibody ratios, little loss of antigen binding by the antibody occurs. However, if loss of binding becomes a problem with a particular antibody, biotin-hydrazide may result in an effective conjugate (see margin note).

Materials
□ affinity-purified anti-glucose oxidase antibody (Step 6, Experiment 5,II)

□ Sulfo-NHS-LC-biotin (Pierce #21335D) [For a less water-soluble version, use NHS-CA-biotin (Pierce # 21336 D; Sigma # B2643).]

□ PBS (Appendix B)

□ 1 M potassium carbonate, pH 8.9

□ dimethylformamide, purged with N_2 for 20–30 min to rid of dimethylamine

□ Sephadex G-50 or dialysis tubing (see Step 3)

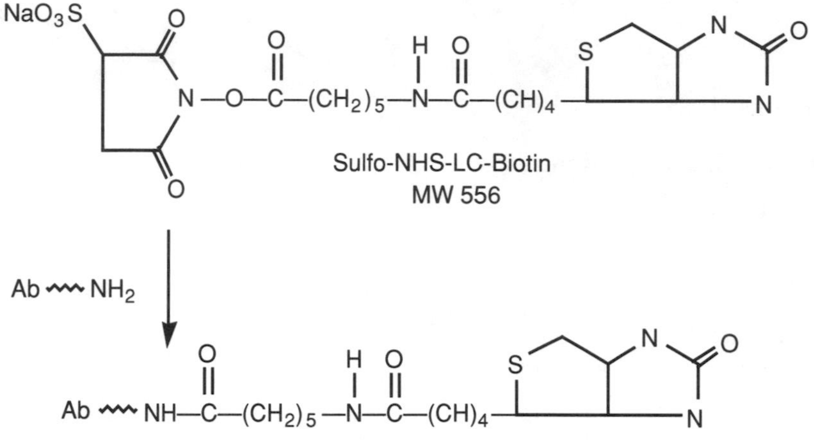

Sulfo-NHS-LC-Biotin
MW 556

FIGURE 6-4

Biotin coupling to antibody.

Biotin-hydrazide will bind to periodate-oxidized antibodies. Sodium periodate generates aldehydes from vicinal diols on the carbohydrate groups of antibodies. Biotin-hydrazide then forms hydrazone linkages with these aldehydes. The resultant conjugate has no biotin near the antibody binding sites, and may show increased antigen binding compared with NHS-biotin derivatives (O'Shannessy and Quarles, 1987).

The biotin analog shown in Figure 6.4 features both an extension arm (LC) and a charged succinimidyl ester (sulfo-NHS). The extension arm promotes stronger binding of the biotin–antibody complex to streptavidin by reducing steric hindrance, whereas the sulfo group promotes water solubility of the biotin analog during conjugation to antibody.

II. Biotin Labeling of Antibody

Procedure

This procedure is a modification of that of Leary *et al.* (1983).

DAY ONE

1. For every 1 ml antibody (0.1–10 mg/ml) in 0.15 M NaCl, add 0.1 ml 1 M carbonate buffer, pH 8.9.

2. To this solution, add Sulfo-NHS-LC-biotin at a ratio of 0.2 mg biotin for every 1 mg antibody. To do this, dissolve biotin in dimethylformamide (DMF) at 5 mg/ml; then add an aliquot of this solution to the antibody to give 0.2 mg biotin for every 1 mg antibody. Be sure no more than 50 μl DMF is added per 1 ml antibody solution; otherwise denaturation of antibody may occur. Allow to react for 1 hr at room temperature.

3. Separate unreacted biotin by dialysis against PBS or by gel filtration through Sephadex G-50. (Use the procedure in Step 7 of the HRP conjugation protocol.)

4. Store biotin–antibody with 0.1% sodium azide at 4°C up to 2 wk, or freeze in aliquots at –70°C for months.

REFERENCES

Avrameas, S. (1969). Coupling of enzymes to proteins with glutaraldehyde. Use of the conjugates for the detection of antigens and antibodies. *Immunochemistry* **6**, 43–52.

Avrameas, S., Ternynck, T., and Guesdon, J.-L. (1979). Coupling of enzymes to antibodies and antigens. *Scand. J. Immunol.* **8**, 7–23.

Bayer, E. A., and Wilchek, M. (1980). The use of the avidin–biotin complex as a tool in molecular biology. *Meth. Biochem. Anal.* **26**, 1–45.

Engvall, E., and Perlman, P. (1971). Enzyme-linked immunosorbent assay (ELISA): Quantitative assay of immlunoglobulin G. *Immunochemistry* **8**, 871–879.

Green, N. M. (1990). Avidin and streptavidin. *Meth. Enzymol.* **184**, 51–67.

Leary, J. J., Brigati, D. J., and Ward, D. C. (1983). Rapid and sensitive colorimetric method for visualizing biotin-labeled DNA probes hybridized to DNA or RNA immobilized on nitrocellulose: Bio-blots. *Proc. Natl. Acad. Sci. U.S.A.* **80**, 4045–4049.

Nakane, P. (1979). Preparation and standardization of enzyme-labeled congugates. *In* "Immunoassays in the Clinical Laboratory" (R. M. Nakamura, W. R. Dito, and E. S. Tucher III, eds.), p. 81–87. Liss, New York.

O'Shannessy, D. J., and Quarles, R. H. (1987). Labeling of the oligosaccharide moieties of immunoglobulins. *J. Immunol. Meth.* **99**, 153–161.

O'Sullivan, M. J., and Marks, V. (1981). Methods for the preparation of enzyme–antibody conjugates for use in enzyme immunoassay. *Meth. Enzymol.* **73**, 147–166.

O'Sullivan, M. J., Gnemmi, E., Morris, D., Chieregatti, G., Simmons, A. D., Simmons, M., Bridges, J. W., and Marks, V. (1979). Comparison of two methods of preparing enzyme–antibody conjugates and application of these conjugates for enzyme immunoassay. *Anal. Biochem.* **100**, 100–108.

Voller, A., Bidwell, D., and Bartlett, A. (1980). Enzyme-linked immunosorbent assay. *In* "Manual of Clinical Immunology", (N. R. Rose and H. Friedman, eds.) p. 359–371, American Society for Microbiology, Washington, D.C.

Wilchek, M., and Bayer, E. A. (1988). The avidin–biotin complex in bioanalytical applications. *Anal. Biochem.* **171**, 1–32.

Protein Blotting

Unpurified test samples often contain many different proteins, making it impossible to measure a single specific protein by chemical assay. Further, the enzymatic or binding properties of the single protein may not be measurable because of interference by other substances in the sample. Although partial separation of proteins in a sample may be obtained with gel electrophoresis, chemical stains detect all proteins in a gel pattern, not a specific protein. Thus, to detect a specific protein in a gel pattern, immunochemical detection is often necessary. This experiment presents the theory and protocol for identifying a single protein in a test sample by electrophoresis and immunochemical detection.

Western or Immunoblotting

To improve the detection of proteins on gels, researchers began to use antibodies to probe the gel patterns. These techniques were hampered both by the need for extensive incubations and washings and by the tendency of gels to tear easily. Development of procedures to transfer proteins from gels to nitrocellulose membranes addressed these difficulties (Towbin *et al.*, 1979; for reviews, see Gershoni and Palade, 1983; Stott, 1989) following the success Southern had with DNA transfers from agarose to nitrocellulose ("Southern blotting;" Southern, 1975). The term "Western blotting" was given to the transfer and immunodetection of *proteins* from gels (Burnette, 1981). Western blotting, also known as immunoblotting, is used to detect the presence and molecular weight of antigens in a crude mixture, to compare immunological cross-reactivity among proteins, and to study modifications of proteins during cellular synthesis. The advantages of using membranes as a substrate for protein detection are ease of membrane manipulation, reduced washing and reaction times, possible reuse of the blot for two or more procedures after removal of probing reagents with detergents or pH shifts, and storage of blots for months before their use. Further, blots are compatible with a variety of detection procedures other than immunochemical, including direct protein dye staining, autoradiography, colorimetric enzyme assays, and ligand binding assays. Typically, proteins may be detected in the nanogram range by one or more of these techniques.

In Western blotting, the protein sample first is separated by SDS–PAGE, then is transferred electrophoretically onto a suitable membrane, and finally detected by a labeled antibody (Figure 7.1). Several aspects of the Western blotting technique deserve comment.

Transfer Procedure

Proteins may be absorbed directly from the gel onto the membrane by simple contact, forcing the proteins to flow into the membrane using vacuum or dry paper. However, these procedures may be ineffective with certain proteins or may take considerable time. Most transfers are accomplished by electrophoresis of the proteins from the gel onto the membrane. Transfer buffers are of low ionic strength, allowing electrophoresis without high currents that generate heat. Methanol often is added to the buffer to increase binding of proteins to nitrocellu-

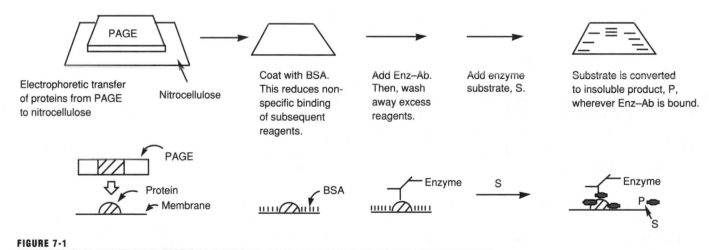

FIGURE 7-1

Western blotting with enzyme-labeled antibody.

lose and to reduce swelling of the gel during transfer. However, methanol reduces the elution of high molecular weight proteins from the gel and requires long times (>12 hr) for efficient transfer.

Types of Membranes

Various types of membrane material are available, each with different advantages. Nitrocellulose is probably the most widely used membrane material, combining ease of use with high binding capacity. New nitrocellulose membranes are available with high tear resistance, overcoming the brittleness of the original nitrocellulose membranes. Nylon membranes are used if hydrophobic proteins are to be bound, but they have lower binding capacity than nitrocellulose. Polyvinylidene difluoride (PVDF) membranes have high capacity and are mechanically stable, but are slightly more troublesome than nitrocellulose or nylon to prepare for transfer. Although all these membranes bind proteins noncovalently, chemically modified papers have been used to covalently bind transferred proteins. Diazobenzyloxymethyl (DBM) and diazophenylthioether (DPT) modified papers bind proteins by diazo linkages, but they are coarser in texture, have limited storage life, and cannot be used with some of the common transfer buffers that contain glycine.

Antibody for Use in Western Blotting

Western blots often are used to detect very minor antigens in a mixture containing many other proteins. For an antibody to detect these minor antigens effectively, it must have a high specificity and a high binding constant ($10^8 - 10^{10}$ M^{-1}). Thus, antibodies with lower binding constants may work well in precipitation techniques in agar gels, but may be unsuitable for Western blotting. Further, since antigens are denatured during SDS–PAGE before transferring to a membrane, an antibody probably recognizes denatured rather than native antigen on the blot. This means that linear rather than conformational epitopes probably are recognized on blots.

Polyclonal and monoclonal antibodies both may be used for blotting, and each has advantages. Polyclonals are often most available and usually have high affinity for the antigen, but they also contain nonspecific antibodies against unknown antigens that may be present in a crude mixture, especially if the mixture is of microbial origin. For this reason, many polyclonals are affinity purified for cleanest results. Monoclonals may be very specific for an antigen and produce minimal background, but their affinity may be low unless they are chosen for high affinity during clone selection. Thus, a *mixture* of monoclonals may combine high affinity with low background ideally.

Labels to Detect the Antigen

Radionuclides and enzymes are the most widely used labels in immunoblotting, but colloidal gold is an alternative (Brada and Roth, 1984; Hsu, 1984). Enzyme labels are faster and more convenient than radiolabels, but they cannot be used to quantitate relative amounts of antigen dependably, and the colored bands generated by the enzymes fade on storage. Radiolabels require more steps to visualize, but they allow quantitation of antigen bands by densitometry or direct counting, and they are capable of generating multiple exposures on films.

Enzyme and radiolabels may be used on a primary antibody or on a secondary molecule. A labeled *primary* antibody localizes directly to the protein on the blot (see Figure 7.1), whereas a labeled *secondary* molecule localizes to an unlabeled primary antibody bound to the protein on the blot (see Figure 7.2). A secondary labeled molecule may be advantageous for a number of reasons: it allows crude antiserum to be used as the unlabeled primary antibody, it often produces an amplification of the antibody–antigen interaction because of the build-up of many layers of labeled molecules, and it reduces the need to label many different primary antibodies. However, a secondary label does require additional steps during the blotting procedure. The most common secondary molecules are anti-immunoglobulin, streptavidin, and protein A. Many labeled secondary molecules are available commercially.

I. Dot Blotting

Dot blots provide an easy semiquantitative immunoassay to detect the presence of an antigen. Samples containing antigen are dotted on a membrane, probed with labeled antibody, and developed (Figure 7.3). No separation on PAGE is done, so the dot blots only provide information about the presence of antigen, not its molecular weight. Estimation of antigen concentration is possible if known standards are

Although SDS is used to denature the proteins in SDS–PAGE, when preparing samples for dot blots SDS should not be included in the buffer. SDS significantly reduces the sensitivity of the dot blots, and the results do not correlate well with proteins transferred from SDS–PAGE gels.

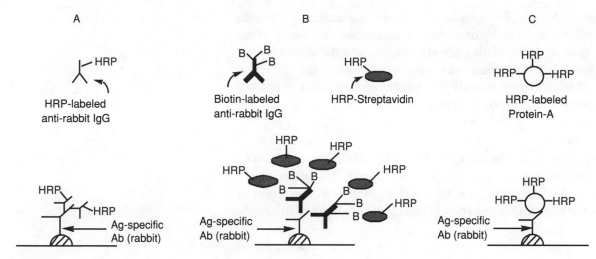

FIGURE 7.2

Immunoblotting with three different secondary molecules. (A) HRP-labeled anti-immunoglobulin.
(B) Biotin-labeled anti-immunoglobulin with HRP–streptavidin. (C) HRP–protein A.

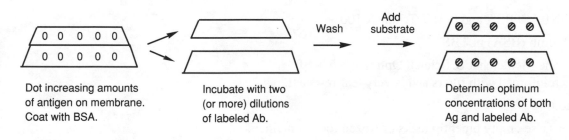

| Dot increasing amounts of antigen on membrane. Coat with BSA. | Incubate with two (or more) dilutions of labeled Ab. | Determine optimum concentrations of both Ag and labeled Ab. |

FIGURE 7.3

Dot blot.

included on the blots, although the blots never provide the accuracy of other immunoassays because of the difficulty of accurately measuring the density of the color. However, the ease of manipulating the membranes and the ability to test many samples simultaneously have made this a popular technique for screening. Dot blots also are used to determine quickly the optimal concentration of antigen and labeled antibody to be used in a Western blot.

Experiment

In the first part of this experiment, dot blots will be used to estimate the amount of labeled anti-glucose oxidase needed to detect glucose oxidase. The use of a secondary label to amplify the detection also will be investigated. The second part of the experiment describes use of a Western blot to detect glucose oxidase in a crude mixture.

Materials

- □ HRP- and biotin-labeled anti-glucose oxidase (Experiment 6)
- □ HRP–streptavidin, (Zymed Laboratories # 43-4323), diluted 1/2000 in TBT buffer
- □ glucose oxidase (Sigma #G7016), diluted to 10, 50, 200, 500, and 1000 µg/ml in TBS
- □ bovine serum, diluted 1/1000, 1/500, 1/100, 1/50, and 1/10 in TBS
- □ TBS (Appendix B)
- □ TBT buffer: TBS with 0.1% BSA and 0.01% Triton-X 100
- □ 2% bovine serum albumin (BSA) in TBS
- □ nitrocellulose membrane (Schleicher & Schuell Optibind # 62940)
  This membrane is reinforced with fibers and is very tear resistant.
- □ capillary tubes for dotting
- □ shallow plastic dishes (Use empty pipet tip racks or frozen food containers approximately 15 × 15 cm on the bottom.)
- □ 4 50-ml screw-capped plastic conical centrifuge tubes
- □ reciprocating shaker (optional)

Procedure

DAY ONE

1. Rule off a 4 × 6-rectangle of nitrocellulose membrane into approximately 0.5-cm squares with a ball point pen; use the pattern in Figure 7.4. Wear gloves, handle by edges only, and work over clean filter paper or paper towels.

2. Prepare sample dilutions of bovine serum and glucose oxidase in TBS. (See concentrations under *Materials*.) Dot 3–5-mm circles with a capillary tube according to Table 7.1 and Figure 7.4.

3. Allow to air dry about 15 min or until no visible wet spot remains.

4. Coat or *block* the membrane with 25 ml 2% BSA in TBS. To do this, place the membrane in a shallow plastic dish containing the BSA–TBS. Incubate for 10 min at room temperature, shaking gently. Store the blot at 4°C after transferring it to a TBS buffer without BSA.

5. Prepare 25 ml each of 1/500 and 1/5000 dilutions of both HRP-labeled and biotin-labeled anti-glucose oxidase in TBT.

   (A) biotin–anti-glucose oxidase: 1/500

   (B) biotin–anti-glucose oxidase: 1/5000

   (C) HRP–anti-glucose oxidase: 1/500

   (D) HRP–anti-glucose oxidase: 1/5000

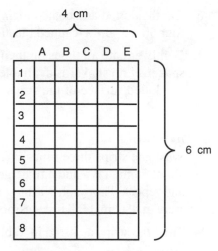

FIGURE 7.4

Set-up for dot blot nitrocellulose membranes.

BSA often is used to block the sites on the membrane not already bound with the dotted sample protein. Other blocking agents include nonfat milk, gelatin, and whole serum from the same species as the primary antibody.

If membranes are stored for extended periods of time in high protein buffers, some displacement of the dotted protein may be caused by the coating or blocking protein.

TABLE 7.1

Samples for Dot Blot Membrane

Strips	Sample	Square A	B	C	D	E
1,3,5,7	Bovine serum (dilution)	1/10	1/50	1/100	1/500	1/1000
2,4,6,8	Glucose oxidase (µg/ml)	1000	500	200	50	10

6. Cut the dotted and coated membrane into strips and divide the strips among four 50-ml screw-capped plastic tubes (see Table 7.2).

7. Gently agitate all tubes on their sides overnight at 4°C on a reciprocating shaker. If no shaker is available, place the tubes on their sides at 4°C with the dotted surface of the strips facing the liquid, not the side of the tube.

DAY TWO

8. Wash the strips three times in TBT. For each wash, suspend the strips in about 25 ml TBT and agitate gently for 1–2 min. Pour off the wash buffer and repeat. Thorough washing reduces background staining. After washing, store at 4°C in TBT if necessary.

   Agitate by gently shaking the strips side to side.

9. Treat the strips as listed in Table 7.3.

10. HRP-containing spots will be visualized using the substrate 4-chloro-1-naphthol, which forms an insoluble purple-grey product with HRP (for procedure, see Appendix D). Dry blots between filter paper and save.

11. Look at all the blots. Choose a concentration of HRP- or biotin-labeled antibody that detects the minimum amount of glucose oxidase and has an acceptable amount of background staining. This concentration of antibody along with the minimum concentration of glucose oxidase will be used to perform the Western blot analysis.

TABLE 7.2
Incubation Conditions for Dot Blots

Strips	Tube number	Anti-glucose Oxidase[a]	
		Biotin-labeled	HRP-labeled
1 and 2	1	1/500	—
3 and 4	2	1/5000	—
5 and 6	3	—	1/500
7 and 8	4	—	1/5000

[a]See Step 5.

TABLE 7.3
Dot Blot Treatment

Strips	Treatment
1 and 2; 3 and 4	Add 25 ml HRP–streptavidin at 1/2000 dilution in TBT; agitate for 1 hr at room temperature, or overnight at 4°C; wash as in Step 8; develop as in Step 10
5 and 6; 7 and 8	Develop according to Step 10

II. Western Blotting

Experiment

Dot blots provide an estimation of antigen and antibody concentration necessary for sensitive low-background blots. In this part of the experiment, these values will be used in a Western blot to detect the presence and molecular weight of glucose oxidase in both crude and pure samples.

Materials

- ☐ HRP- or biotin-labeled anti-glucose oxidase at optimum concentration for probing blots, determined from dot blot; dilute in TBT buffer
- ☐ bovine serum, diluted 1/50 in TBS as a negative control (no glucose oxidase)
- ☐ glucose oxidase, crude (Sigma #G6766), 1 mg/ml in TBS
- ☐ glucose oxidase, pure (Sigma #G7016), at a concentration determined by dot blot, Step 11; dilute in TBS buffer
- ☐ unknown glucose oxidase samples consisting of varying amounts of glucose oxidase mixed with other proteins or bovine serum
- ☐ TBS (Appendix B)
- ☐ 2% BSA in TBS buffer
- ☐ plastic wrap
- ☐ *n*-butanol
- ☐ power supply
- ☐ slab gel apparatus with tank, sandwich, spacers, and combs
- ☐ boiling water bath or 100°C heating block
- ☐ Hamilton syringe or micropipet
- ☐ transfer buffer (Appendix D)
- ☐ nitrocellulose membrane

☐ electrotransfer apparatus (e.g. BioRad "Trans-Blot"; Hoeffer "TE42")

☐ filter paper cut to fit transfer sandwich (Appendix D)

☐ Scotch Brite pads to fit transfer sandwich (Appendix D)

Procedure

DAY ONE

1. Prepare samples of standard proteins, bovine serum, and glucose oxidase at concentrations determined from the dot blots. Consult with the instructor. Electrophorese samples on SDS–PAGE (Appendix C). A suggested PAGE might be:

   1. Standard proteins

   2. Bovine serum

   3. Glucose oxidase

   4. Bovine serum

   5. Glucose oxidase

   6–10. Unknown mixtures of glucose oxidase and other proteins

   After electrophoresis on SDS–PAGE, the separated proteins will be transferred, or "blotted," to a nitrocellulose membrane. Lanes 1–3 will be stained for total protein using amido black, whereas lanes 4 and 5 will be "probed" with the labeled anti-glucose oxidase to determine the molecular weight and presence of glucose oxidase in bovine serum. Additional lanes 6–10 may be probed with the antibody to determine glucose oxidase in an unknown mixture.

   The instructors will demonstrate how to sandwich the PAGE gel next to the nitrocellulose membrane and will transfer the proteins to the membrane electrophoretically overnight. (See Appendix D for details on these procedures.) The membrane blot is now ready to be visualized.

DAY TWO

2. Cut lanes 1–3 from the blot in one strip. To do this, place the blot on top of a fresh sheet of parafilm and cut with a razor blade. Stain with amido black (Appendix D).

3. While performing Step 2, coat the remainder of the blot with 2% BSA in TBS for 15 min in a shallow plastic tray. Next, add the optimal concentration of either HRP- or biotin-labeled anti-glucose oxidase, as determined from the dot blot results. Use TBT as a diluent.

4. Incubate 6–48 hr at 4°C with shaking.

DAY THREE

5. When using the biotin-labeled anti-glucose oxidase, an additional incubation with HRP–streptavidin (1/2000 or dilution suggested by supplier) for 1 hr at room temperature is required. Wash four times between the biotin anti-glucose oxidase incubation and the HRP–streptavidin addition.

6. Wash blot four times with TBT.

7. Develop blot with chloronapthol (Appendix D).

Questions

1. Which samples contain glucose oxidase, according to the Western blot? Does this correspond to expected results?

2. Are there other bands detected by antibody in the unknown samples? Why are these visualized? What parameters (e.g., Ab or Ag concentration) could be changed to reduce these bands?

3. What control could be run to provide evidence that the anti-glucose oxidase detected glucose oxidase, not another protein with identical molecular weight?

4. What is the minimum mass of glucose oxidase detected on the Western blot? Does the molecular weight of the glucose oxidase correspond to literature values?

REFERENCES

Brada, D., and Roth, J. (1984). "Golden blot"—Detection of polyclonal and monoclonal antibodies bound to antigens on nitrocellulose by protein-A–gold complexes. *Anal. Biochem.* **142**, 79–83.

Burnette, W. N. (1981). "Western Blotting": Electrophoretic transfer of proteins from sodium dodecyl sulfate-polyacrylamide gels to unmodified nitrocellulose and radiographic detection with antibody and radioiodinated protein A. *Anal. Biochem.* **112**, 195–203.

Danscher, G. and Norgaard, J. O. R. (1983). Light microscopic visualization of colloidal gold on resin-embedded tissue. *J. Histochem. Cytochem.* **31**, 1394–1398.

Gershoni, J. M., and Palade, G. E. (1983). Protein blotting: Principles and applications. *Anal. Biochem.* **134**, 1–15.

Hsu, Y.-H. (1984). Immunogold for detection of antigen on nitrocellulose paper. *Anal. Biochem.* **142**, 221–225.

Southern, E. M. (1975). Detection of specific sequences among DNA fragments separated by gel electrophoresis. *J. Mol. Biol.* **98**, 503–517.

Stott, D. I. (1989). Immunoblotting and dot blotting. *J. Immunol. Meth.* **119**, 153–187.

Towbin, H., Staehelin, T., and Gordon, J. (1979). Electrophoretic transfer of proteins from polyacrylamide gels to nitrocelluose sheets: procedure and some applications. *Proc. Natl. Acad. Sci. U.S.A.* **76**, 4350–4354.

Immunoprecipitation with Staphylococcal Protein A

Many proteins occur in very small amounts in cell extracts, making it difficult to determine their presence and molecular weight. Immunoprecipitation, first introduced by Kessler (Kessler, 1975; Ivarie and Jones, 1979) has enabled scientists to analyze such proteins. In this technique, an antibody to a specific protein is added to a cell extract, forming an antibody–antigen complex. The complex is then removed from the bulk of the contaminants in the extract by adsorption onto solid-phase *Staphylococcus aureus* protein A (see Experiment 5). Finally, the antigen is analyzed by any number of electrophoretic, enzymatic, or radioisotopic procedures.

In this experiment, immunoprecipitation will be used to detect both radiolabeled and unlabeled glucose oxidase from a protein mixture. Because immunoprecipitation is an extremely powerful and versatile technique, a theoretical discussion will be presented first.

BASIC PROTOCOL USED IN IMMUNOPRECIPITATION

The most common immunoprecipitation procedure uses radiolabeled cells. It has four steps.

1. First, a cell extract is radiolabeled, either by prior biosynthetic incorporation of a radiolabeled precursor or by chemical radiolabeling following preparation of the extract. During either procedure, all proteins in the extract are radiolabeled.

2. Second, a primary antibody is added that binds to a specific antigen of interest. The antibody is added in excess, so all the antigen is bound in a soluble antibody–antigen complex.

3. Third, this complex is separated from other tissue proteins by adsorption to a solid-phase form of protein A. Protein A binds to the antibody in the complex and retains it on the solid phase as an immunoprecipitate. The immunoprecipitate is washed repeatedly by centrifugation to remove contaminating proteins.

4. Finally, the antigen (radiolabeled) is released from the antibody and Protein A by boiling in SDS. The released antigen is then electrophoresed on SDS–PAGE and detected by autoradiography (placing the gel against a photographic film and allowing the radioactive antigen to expose the film).

Immunoprecipitation combines the exquisite specificity of an antibody to bind its antigen with the ability of protein A to remove the antibody–antigen complex from a crude mixture. Thus, almost any antigen is subject to analysis by this method, as long as a suitable antibody is available. It is an exceptionally powerful technique, because even nonprecipitating antigens such as small peptides may be studied. An added advantage is that immunoprecipitation can concentrate trace antigens from a large volume of sample.

Analysis of Immunoprecipitated Antigen

By far the most common analysis of an immunoprecipitated antigen is determination of molecular weight after Western blotting. In this procedure, both the relative amounts of antigen in different tissue samples and the size of the antigen after metabolic processing can be determined. If the antigen is not analyzed by Western blotting, it can be released from protein A with either SDS or high salts and can be subjected to chemical or enzymatic treatments to study function or structure (e.g., carbohydrate analysis of lipase; Doolittle *et al.*, 1990).

CRITICAL ASPECTS OF IMMUNOPRECIPITATION

Types of Solid-Phase Protein A Used for Adsorption

Protein A occurs on the surface of certain staphylococci and binds the Fc portion of many immunoglobulin isotypes. Two forms of protein A normally are used in immunoprecipitation: formalin fixed cells of *Staphylococcus aureus* (Staph A) that retain active protein A on their surfaces, or protein A–agarose that has purified protein A bound covalently (see Experiment 5). Although fixed Staph A cells are less expensive and have a higher capacity than protein A–agarose, they may bind nonspecific proteins from crude mixtures more readily than the protein A–agarose. These nonspecific proteins will result in additional bands after blotting and may be confused with the immunospecific bands. For this reason, fixed Staph A preparations may require extensive washing in either SDS or nonionic detergents to remove interfering substances that promote spurious binding. Both types of adsorbants are available commercially and, ultimately, both types must be tested to determine the one most effective for a specific experiment.

Radiolabeling Cells

Cells to be used for immunoprecipitation may be radiolabeled either by metabolic incorporation of ^{35}S or by chemical labeling with ^{125}I or ^{3}H. The ^{35}S isotope has a relatively short half-life (87 days) and is detected easily by a gamma counter or by autoradiography (Bonifacino, 1991). If only the cell-surface proteins are to be labeled, then whole cells may be treated with ^{125}I and lactoperoxidase (which labels surface tyrosines; Samelson, 1991) or with ^{3}H and borohydride reduction (which labels surface carbohydrate). Both methods are gentle enough to insure little denaturing of surface proteins.

Preparation of Tissue Extracts

Cellular antigens include those that are soluble and those that are membrane bound inside the cell. Both types of antigens must be dissociated from their environment by rupturing the membranes and releasing the antigens in a form recognized by the antibody. For cytosolic proteins, simple release from the interior by homogenization may suffice, but for membrane-bound antigens the membrane must be dissociated effectively to insure complete release of the antigen.

Membrane dissolution normally is accomplished by a detergent, which serves two functions. First, the detergent dissolves the membrane (plasma membrane, mitochondrial membrane, or nuclear membrane) by incorporating the membrane lipids into detergent micelles. Second, the detergent must surround the hydrophobic areas on the antigen and solubilize it away from the membrane. If the proper detergent is chosen, the membrane antigen is released in a soluble form that is available for binding by specific antibody. Normally, a combination of both physical homogenization and the presence of a detergent is required for efficient antigen release.

Different detergents are used for cell lysis, from the highly denaturing ionic detergents such as SDS and cetyltrimethylammonium bromide to the mildly denaturing sodium deoxycholate and popular nonionic polyoxyethylene-based detergents such as Triton X-100 and Brij 58 (see Appendix I) (Hjellmeland, 1990; Neugebauer, 1990). The detergent concentration necessary for antigen release varies among tissues and antigens, but in all cases the detergent used must still allow effective antibody–antigen binding. Once again, empirical determination of the optimum detergent must be done to insure effective antigen release and subsequent antibody binding.

Usually, 1–3% nonionic detergents are tried first to release a membrane antigen, then, 0.1–0.5% ionic detergents. Nonionic detergents rarely interfere with antibody binding, but ionic detergents often interfere. If an ionic detergent such as SDS is necessary to release antigen, a 5–10-fold excess of a nonionic detergent (e.g., Triton X-100) may be added after membrane dissolution to bind excess ionic detergent and allow effective antibody binding in the subsequent immunoprecipitation step.

Requirements for Antibodies Used in Immunoprecipitation

An antibody must have high affinity ($>10^7$ M^{-1}) and narrow specificity to be effective in immunoprecipitation. Antibodies with lower binding constants may be useful for detecting antigens that occur in high concentrations, but may not detect antigens that occur in low concentrations. Thus, an antibody that performs well in an Ouchterlony precipitation test, which does not require a high affinity antibody, may not work in immunoprecipitation techniques.

Both polyclonal and monoclonal antibodies may be effective in immunoprecipitation. Polyclonal antibodies are often of high affinity as a result of extensive boosting during immunization. This high affinity, along with their multivalent nature, often allows polyclonals to form large specific antibody–antigen complexes that bind very effectively to protein A. Monoclonals normally have lower affinity than polyclonals, but they often have considerably less interference, both because they bind only one epitope (and rarely cross-react with other antigens) and because they contain no other antibodies. Further, monoclonals may be elicited against an impure antigen, a procedure impossible with polyclonals, by immunizing mice with a crude preparation of the antigen, using the animal to create a panel of hybridomas, and finally selecting a clone that produces a mono-clonal specific for the antigen. Thus, a mixture of high affinity monoclonals that have different epitope specificities for the same antigen may combine the best fea-tures of both kinds of antibody preparations, but is difficult to produce.

Finally, an antibody must be bound tightly by protein A for effective immuno-precipitation. If a primary antibody against an antigen does not bind well to pro-tein A, then a secondary antibody may be added that does bind well to protein A. Rabbit antibody against the Fc region of the primary antibody is used often since it binds protein A strongly.

Methods to Reduce Background Interference during Immunoprecipitation

Proteins other than the antigen occur in the immunoprecipitates for two reasons: they bind to the antibody or they bind nonspecifically to the solid-phase protein A. Since the antibody is chosen to optimize antigen binding (see previous section), nonspecific binding to the solid-phase protein A is the most prevalent cause of spurious protein binding.

A number of procedures are used to reduce nonspecific binding to protein A. First, protein A–agarose appears to have fewer sites for nonspecific binding than fixed Staph A. Simply switching to this solid phase may help considerably. Second, buffers that incorporate both nonionic detergents (Triton X-100, NP-40) and high concentrations of carrier protein (serum albumin, gelatin) may reduce nonspecific binding. Third, the solid-phase protein A may be pretreated with an *unlabeled* tissue extract before exposure to the *radiolabeled* extract . Nonspecific sites on the protein A will be filled primarily with unlabeled protein which will not appear as bands on autoradiograms. Fourth, prior to adding antibody, the cell extract may be pretreated with solid-phase protein A to absorb any nonspecific proteins (Firestone and Winguth, 1990). Fifth, after immunoprecipitation, the anti-body–antigen complex may be dissociated from protein A with SDS, and adsorbed back onto fresh protein A. The nonspecifically bound proteins are removed along with the old protein A (Platt *et al.*, 1986).

ALTERNATIVE PRECIPITATION AND LABELING PROCEDURES

Alternatives to Protein A for Immunoprecipitation

There are methods other than using protein A to remove antibody–antigen complexes from a sample. For instance, a secondary antibody against the primary antibody may be used to precipitate the original antibody–antigen complex. However, because minuscule amounts of primary antibody are used to bind antigen, *nonspecific* antibody from the same species as the primary antibody must be added to increase the volume of the primary antibody. This insures that sufficiently large complexes will form and precipitate. Another method incorporates biotinylated primary antibody to form the antibody–antigen complexes, which then may be adsorbed onto streptavidin–agarose (Kern *et al.*, 1990).

Alternatives to Radiolabeling

Detection of a cellular antigen without using radiolabeled cell samples is also possible. In one procedure, antigen first is immunoprecipitated with antibody and solid-phase protein A, electrophoresed, and blotted onto a membrane. Next, the membrane is treated with antigen-specific antibody, which binds to corresponding antigen bands on the membranes. After a wash step, labeled protein A is added, which binds to the immobilized antibody. Thus, a "sandwich" is built on the membrane that contains (in order) antigen, antibody, and labeled protein A. This procedure obviates radiolabeling of cells and allows the researcher to choose radioisotope- or enzyme-labeled protein A to detect antigen. However, this technique does require a number of additional steps, and the primary antibody must be capable of detecting antigen (after SDS–PAGE) adsorbed to nitrocellulose.

Alternatively, labeled anti-Fc antibody may be used instead of protein A to bind the antigen-specific antibody.

Experiment

In this experiment, two different methods will be used to detect radiolabeled glucose oxidase or unlabeled glucose oxidase after immunoprecipitation. To begin, Staph A will be used to immunoprecipitate an antibody–glucose oxidase complex; the precipitate will be used for SDS–PAGE and blotting to nitrocellulose membrane. One method will use autoradiography to detect radiolabeled glucose oxidase; the other method will use enzyme-labeled antibody to detect unlabeled glucose oxidase.

Materials

Common materials needed for both detection methods

□ rabbit anti-glucose oxidase serum.

If only goat or sheep antiserum is available, rabbit anti-goat (or sheep) IgG is necessary. Goat and sheep antisera are bound poorly by Staph A (see Experiment 5). If these species are the antiserum source, then rabbit anti-goat (or sheep) IgG must be included to provide a secondary antibody to which Staph A will bind (see Step 4).

□ control serum, same species as anti-glucose oxidase serum

□ glucose oxidase, 1 mg/ml (as a standard for the Western blot)

□ protein mixture, containing 1 mg/ml each glucose oxidase, ovalbumin, and carbonic anhydrase, and 0.20 mg/ml bovine serum albumin.

This is a synthetic protein mixture designed to mimic partly a crude extract from which glucose oxidase will be immunoprecipitated. Because BSA iodinates and stains more readily than the other proteins, it must be used at a lower concentration to approximate equal detection among all proteins. Alternatively, serum may be "spiked" with glucose oxidase. Crude lysates of *aspergillus niger*, the source species for glucose oxidase, are ideal for immunoprecipitation, but are difficult to obtain commercially. However, many microbiology departments have cultures of *A. niger* as a source from which to prepare crude lysates.

☐ Staph A, 10% suspension (formalin-fixed *Staphylococcus aureus*; Sigma #P7155)

Wash 200 μl of the suspension in wash buffer shortly before use. For critical procedures, the Staph A may have to be washed extensively in 1% Triton X-100 or 0.1% SDS to remove surface material that binds proteins nonspecifically.

☐ wash buffer: 0.15 M NaCl, 0.010 M Tris, 0.005 M EDTA, 0.10% Triton X-100, pH 7.4

☐ 1 M sucrose in wash buffer

☐ PAGE sample preparation buffer (SPB; Appendix C)

☐ PAGE apparatus and reagents (Appendix C)

☐ electrotransfer apparatus

☐ Western blotting reagents (Appendix D)

Additional materials needed for ^{125}I-labeled glucose oxidase detection

☐ ^{125}I-labeled mixture of proteins, including 1 mg/ml each glucose oxidase, ovalbumin, carbonic anhydrase, and 0.1 mg/ml bovine serum albumin.

This is a synthetic "crude" protein mixture from which glucose oxidase will be immunoprecipitated. 10 μl of this mixture is labeled with 0.5 mCi of carrier-free Na^{125}I (Amersham #IMS.30) by the chloramine-T procedure (Appendix I). An appropriate activity is $1–10 \times 10^4$ cpm/μl ($1–10 \times 10^6$ cpm/μg total protein). Alternatively, a serum sample may be "spiked" with glucose oxidase and then radiolabeled, but the albumin becomes the dominant protein labeled and sensitivity is decreased, resulting in longer autoradiograph exposure times. Crude lysates of *Aspergillus niger* are difficult to obtain commercially but are ideal mixtures for iodination.

☐ X-ray film for autoradiography [X-OMAT-AR or X-OMAT-RP film (Kodak, Sigma) or Hyperfilm-MP (Amersham)]

□ exposure cassettes.

These cassettes should have an intensifying screen such as DuPont Cronex Lightning Plus (Sigma) or Hyperscreen (Amersham) and be able to withstand a temperature of −70°C.

□ developing chemicals for film [Kodak GBX developer and fixer (Sigma)]

Additional materials needed for unlabeled glucose oxidase detection

□ enzyme-labeled or biotin-labeled anti-glucose oxidase (Experiment 6)

Procedure

DAY ONE

1. To each of two 1.5-ml microfuge tubes, numbered 1S and 2S, add 25 μl ^{125}I-labeled protein mixture (if ^{125}I detection is to be used) or 25 μl *unlabeled* protein mixture diluted 1/100 in wash buffer (if enzyme detection is to be used). Add 25 μl wash buffer to both tubes.

2. To tube 1S, add 10 μl anti-glucose oxidase. To tube 2S, add 10 μl control serum (nonspecific control).

3. Incubate both tubes at 37°C for 15 min, then at 0°C for 15 min (or overnight).

DAY TWO

4. If *rabbit* anti-glucose oxidase was used in Step 2, proceed directly to Step 5. If *goat* or *sheep* anti-glucose oxidase was used in Step 2, then 40 μl (approximately 4-fold excess) of rabbit anti-goat (or sheep) IgG is added to the samples and incubated for an additional 30 min.

5. Add 25 μl 10 % Staph A suspension (previously washed once in wash buffer), vortex, and incubate at 37°C for 30 min with gentle mixing every 10 min to keep the Staph A suspended.

6. Prepare two microfuge tubes, numbered 1P and 2P, each containing 500 μl 1 M sucrose in wash buffer.

CAUTION! All manipulations with ^{125}I must be done with gloves over absorbent leak-proof paper. Proper safety precautions and waste disposal must be observed for the handling of ^{125}I. Follow the directions of the instructor.

Affinity purified anti-glucose oxidase may be included in an additional tube for comparison with whole serum.

The amount of rabbit anti-IgG to use depends on the strength of the antiserum. To optimize this reagent, varying amounts of rabbit anti-IgG should be added to identical sample tubes to determine which amount maximally immunoprecipitates primary antibody.

7. Using a 100–200 μl micropipet, carefully remove all the suspension from tube 1S and gently layer it on top of the 1P sucrose pad. *Be gentle with these tubes to prevent mixing the sucrose and the Staph A mixture!* Repeat for tubes 2S and 2P. Discard tubes 1S and 2S in radioactive waste.

8. Microfuge 1P and 2P for 3 min to pellet the Staph A. Remove all supernatant, sucrose included, *but be careful not to disturb the Staph A pellet!* Use a micropipet to remove the supernatant in a number of repeat suctions. Discard supernatant in radioactive waste.

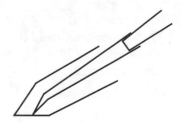

Bend the micropipet tip to remove the supernatant effectively.

9. Add 50 μl wash buffer to each tube, vortex to suspend the Staph A, then add an additional 0.5–1.0 ml wash buffer. Mix well and microfuge for 2–3 min to pellet the Staph A. Remove supernatant as completely as possible and discard in radioactive waste.

The first 50 μl promotes efficient vortexing and suspension of the Staph A.

10. Prepare 250 μl PAGE *reducing* sample preparation buffer diluted 1:4 with water (1 part 4X SPB, 3 parts water). Add 25 μl of this diluted SPB to each Staph A pellet; stir with the pipet tip to resuspend the pellet thoroughly.

11. Cap the tube, prick the top with a 20–25 gauge needle to release pressure, and heat at 37°C for 30 min or at 100°C for 5 min. Cool and keep at –20°C (freezer) until used for SDS–PAGE electrophoresis.

DAY THREE

12. When ready to run the PAGE gel, thaw, vortex, and microfuge the sample for 3 min before applying the *entire* supernatant to the PAGE gel. Apply supernatants from tubes 1P and 2P to the PAGE gel, along with the samples suggested. Electrophorese and transfer to nitrocellulose membrane as described in Experiment 7 and Appendices C and D.

For ¹²⁵I detection (After electrophoresis and transfer, go to Step 13.)

Suggested Patterns for Sample Application to Slots in Gel

1. protein molecular weight standards (apply 1 μg for each band)

2. glucose oxidase standard (apply 1–2 μg)

3. protein mixture (apply 1–2 μg of each protein)

4. ¹²⁵I protein mixture (apply 10 μl)

5. supernatant from tube 1P Staph A pellet

6. supernatant from tube 2P Staph A pellet

For enzyme detection (After electrophoresis and transfer, go to Step 14.)

1. protein molecular weight standards (apply 1 μg each band)

2. glucose oxidase standard (apply 1–2 μg)

3. protein mixture (apply 1–2 μg of each protein)

4. glucose oxidase standard (apply 0.5 μg)

5. protein mixture (apply 0.5 μg of each protein)

6. supernatant from tube 1P Staph A pellet

7. supernatant from tube 2P Staph A pellet

DAY FOUR

13. *For ^{125}I detection of blots*

   a. Stain membrane in amido black (Appendix D). Dry the membrane between sheets of filter paper.

   b. Expose the membrane to X-ray film as follows. Cut two X-ray films slightly larger than the membrane. In a darkroom under red safelight, tape the membrane onto one of the films with one small piece of transparent tape. Be careful not to place the tape over any of the protein bands.

   c. Carefully place a small mark on the film at the corners of the membrane with a fine permanent marker. These marks will enable you to orient the membrane over the film after development.

   d. Open the cassette and insert, in order; one intensifying screen, the film and membrane, another piece of film, another intensifying screen.

   e. Close the cassette tightly and place into a –70°C freezer (–20°C, if –70°C is not available) and expose for 1–2 hr. The low temperature reduces background haze due to autoscintillation of the intensifying screens.

f. Allow the cassette to warm to room temperature so that condensation does not form on the film. In the darkroom under red light, open the cassette and remove the loose film. Close the cassette tightly and develop the film for 1 min in the GBX developer, rinse briefly in water, and fix for 1 min in GBX fixer. Turn on the lights and look for bands on the film. If no bands are evident, or if they are not dark enough, continue exposing the cassette for additional time until the second piece of film is exposed properly. Dry the films in air after a 2–5 min rinse in water.

g. New pieces of film may be exposed as many times as needed to obtain the best images.

14. *For enzyme detection of blots*

a. Cut lanes 1–3 from the membrane and stain in amido black (Appendix D). Place the remaining lanes in 2% BSA with TBS to block further protein absorption to the membrane.

b. Probe the membrane with the optimal concentrations of either enzyme-labeled or biotin-labeled anti-glucose oxidase determined by dot blot analysis in Experiment 7.

Questions

1. Explain the presence of any stained bands seen on the ^{125}I-labeled membrane and film. Are the bands specific for glucose oxidase? How do you know?

2. Did the biotin- or enzyme-labeled antibody detect only glucose oxidase?

3. Calculate the nanograms of glucose oxidase detected by both enzyme and radiolabel detection procedures. Can you determine if one procedure is more sensitive?

4. What could be done to increase the sensitivity of either procedure?

5. In the ^{125}I detection procedure, what creates the extra bands in the immuno-precipitate sample lanes 5 and 6 when stained with amido black?

REFERENCES

Bonifacino, J. S. (1991). Biosynthetic labeling of proteins. *In* "Current Protocols in Immunology" (J. E. Coligan, A. M. Druisbeek, D. H. Margulies, E. M. Shevach, and W. Stober, eds.), pp. 8.12.1–8.12.9. Wiley and Sons, New York.

Doolittle, M. H., Ben-Zeev, O., Elovson, J., Martein, D., and Kirchgessner, T. G. (1990). The response of lipoprotein lipase to feeding and fasting. Evidence for posttranslational regulation. *J. Biol. Chem.* **265**, 4570–4577.

Firestone, G. L., and Winguth, S. D. (1990). Immunoprecipitation of proteins. *Meth. Enzymol.* **182**, 688–700.

Hjelmeland, L. M. (1990). Solubilization of native membrane proteins. *Meth. Enzymol.* **182**, 252–264.

Ivarie, R. D., and Jones, P. P. (1979). A rapid sensitive assay for specific protein synthesis in cells and in cell-free translations: Use of *Staphylococcus aureus* as an adsorbant for immune complexes. *Anal. Biochem.* **97**, 24–35.

Kern, P. A., Martin, R. A., Carty, J., Goldberg, I. J., and Ong, J. M. (1990). Identification of lipoprotein lipase immunoreactive protein in pre- and postheparin plasma from normal subjects and patients with type I hyperlipoproteinemia. *J. Lip. Res.* **31**, 17–26.

Kessler, S. W. (1975). Rapid isolation of antigens from cells with a staphylococcal protein A–antibody adsorbent: Parameters of the interactions of antibody–antigen complexes with protein A. *J. Immunol.* **115**, 1617–1624.

Neugebauer, J. M. (1990). Detergents: An overview. *Meth. Enzymol.* **182**, 239–252.

Platt, E. J., Karlsen, K., Lopez-Valdivieso, A., Cook, P. W., and Firestone, G. L. (1986). Highly sensitive immunoadsorption procedure for detection of low-abundance proteins. *Anal. Biochem.* **156**, 126–135.

Samelson, L. E. (1991). Iodination of soluble and membrane-bound proteins. *In* "Current Protocols in Immunology" (J. E. Coligan, A. M. Druisbeek, D. H. Margulies, E. M. Shevach, and W. Stober, eds.), pp. 8.11.1–8.11.4. Wiley and Sons, New York.

Immunocytochemical Staining of Lymphocytes

The use of antibodies to detect cellular antigens has expanded our knowledge of both the internal structure and the classification of cells greatly. In immunochemical staining of cells, antibodies bind to surface or intracellular antigens and then are detected by one of many labels: enzyme, isotope, fluorophore, or colloidal gold. If the cells are fixed suitably to preserve cell morphology, then the antigens may be localized within the cell and visualized by either electron or light microscopy. Cells in suspension may be passed through a flow cytometer and categorized according to size and distribution of antigen.

In this experiment, surface IgM on mouse lymphocytes will be detected by immunocytochemical methods. Although the assay will be performed on a slide and observed through a light microscope, the principles involved in this experiment may be applied to detection by flow cytometry or electron microscopy also.

Surface Antigens on Lymphocytes

The different subclasses of lymphocytes may be differentiated by antibodies specific for surface proteins. Lymphocyte surface proteins differ depending on the type and number of histocompatibility antigens, the presence or absence of various receptors and channels, and the stage of differentiation or cell growth (Table 9.1) (Bierer and Burakoff, 1988; Knapp *et al.*, 1989; Strominger, 1989; Klein, 1990). Commercial monoclonal antibodies are available against many of the surface antigens and often are used to subdivide lymphocytes into B and T cell subclasses. Analysis of cell populations with these antibodies has enabled scientists to correlate the roles of cell subclasses in the immune response and in disease states.

TABLE 9.1

Common Lymphocyte Cell-Surface Markers[a]

Marker	Cell type[b]	Function	Monoclonal Antibody[c]
CD2	T, NK	red cell receptor; adhesion	Leu 5B, OKT11, T11
CD3	T	TCR signal transducer	Leu4, OKT3, T3
CD4	$T_{helper/inducer}$	MHC II receptor	Leu3, OKT4, T4
CD8	$T_{cytotoxic}$	MHC I receptor	Leu2, OKT8, T8
CD16 (FcγRIII)	NK	Fcγ receptor (low affinity)	Leu11
CD19	B	Part of B-cell antigen receptor?	Leu12, B4
CD20	B	Regulated Ca^{2+} channel?	Leu16, B1
CD21 (CR2)	B	complement C3d receptor; Epstein-Barr virus receptor	CR2, B2
CD25 (Tac, IL-2R)	activated B and T	IL-2 receptor	
CD32 (FcγRII)	activated B	IgG and IgA receptor	
CD35 (CR1)	B	complement C3b receptor	
TCR	T	T cell antigen receptor	

[a]Data from Bieren and Burakoff (1988); Carter and Fearon (1992); Klein (1990); Knapp *et al.* (1989); and Ravetch and Kinet (1991).

[b]T, T cell; B, B cell; NK, natural killer cell.

[c]The Leu and CR series antibodies are available from Becton Dickinson, the OKT series from Ortho Diagnostics, and the T, B series from Coulter-Electronics.

Flow Cytometry

The availability of monoclonal antibodies to many different surface antigens, and the simultaneous development of the flow cytometer, has resulted in a powerful tool to study cell classification (Jackson and Warner, 1986; Shapiro, 1988). In this technique, also known as fluorescence-activated cell sorting (FACS), fluorescently labeled antibodies first are incubated with a cell population. Cells containing the specific antigen on their surface bind the labeled antibody; the cells are diluted extensively before being dispensed from a nozzle in single-cell droplets. The cytometer scans each droplet with an intense (laser) excitation wavelength. If the cell is labeled, it fluoresces, and may be separated, or sorted, by electrostatic deflection. Light given off during the scan is plotted against cell number; the plot is analyzed subsequently to provide limited information about the sizes of the cells and the density of antigens on the surface. Dual beam cytometers provide additional information by scanning for the presence of two different antigens on the same cell. The instruments are very sophisticated and require careful maintenance for optimum results. Therefore, most investigators isolate and label cells with antibody, and then provide a sample to an operator who performs the analysis.

The cytometer largely has supplanted cell staining techniques when information about cell-surface antigens is required. The cytometer offers information about living cells, whereas microscopic techniques necessitate killing and fixing the cells to slides or wire grids with possible masking or alteration of antigens. However, *intracellular* antigens still must be analyzed by microscopy; continuing efforts have improved the quality of antibodies to provide accurate information on histology, cell substructure, and antigen localization.

Microscopic Visualization of Cellular Antigens

Tissue sections and cell suspensions or lysates may be analyzed for the presence of specific antigens by electron and light microscopy. In these techniques, either thin sections of tissues or cells are incubated with antigen-specific primary antibody. The primary antibody then is visualized by a labeled second antibody (or by virtue of a label on the primary antibody). If the label is an enzyme or a gold colloid, an insoluble product is deposited around the antibody–antigen complex, identifying the section of tissue or cell containing the antigen. Alternatively, fluorescently labeled antibody gives off light that is observed in a light microscope, whereas radiolabeled antibody results in the deposition of silver grains visible by light or electron microscopy (Table 9.2) (Winchester and Ross, 1986).

Endogenous peroxidase activity in tissue and cells still may be present after fixation, and may cause false positive staining or high background. Red cells and granulocytes are notorious for causing this problem.

Amplification Techniques for Enzyme Labels

The quality of images obtained by immunocytochemical techniques depends both on the type of label and on the distribution of antigen in the cell. For instance, antigens that are spread in a diffuse pattern over the surface of a cell may be difficult to visualize, even if present in many copies (but a cytometer may still be capable of reading the fluorescence and deflecting such a cell). However, cytoskeletal components often are visualized effectively because the antibody is concentrated on a well-defined structure. Thus, amplification techniques often are used to

TABLE 9.2

Labels Used in Immunocytochemistry

Label	Visible signal	Development	Microscope	Reference
enzyme	insoluble product	enzymatic[a] ABC PAP APAAP	light	Hsu *et al.* (1981) Sternberger (1978) Cordell *et al.* (1984)
radioisotope (^{125}I)	reduced silver in photo emulsion	photo developer	light, electron	
gold colloid	reduced silver surrounds gold	silver reduced from solution	light, electron	Danscher and Norgaard (1983); De Waele *et al.* (1989)
fluorophore	fluorescence	none	light (also FACS)	Winchester and Ross (1986)

[a]Abbreviations: ABC, avidin–biotin–peroxidase; PAP, peroxidase anti-peroxidase; APAAP, alkaline phosphatase anti-alkaline phosphatase.

increase the signal. For enzyme labels, this includes building up multiple copies of labeled secondary molecules (Avidin-Biotin-Peroxidase, ABC; Hsu *et al.*, 1981) or the use of preformed enzyme–antibody complexes that bind the primary antibody (Alkaline Phosphatase Anti-Alkaline Phosphatase, APAAP; Cordell *et al.*, 1984). Gold colloids also may be amplified by depositing silver from enhancement solutions around the gold (Danscher and Norgaard, 1983; De Waele, 1989).

B Lymphocytes, Surface IgM, and Fc Receptors

B cells constitute 10–15% of the circulating lymphocytes and may be detected by the presence of immunoglobulin on their surface. IgM and IgD are embedded in the B cell membrane with a special 25-amino acid "tail" (mIg). These immunoglobulins act as antigen receptors and, when bound with antigen, transfer a signal to the interior of the cell, resulting in growth and proliferation of the B cell into an antibody-producing plasma cell.

B cells also have immunoglobulin bound to their surface by *receptor* molecules. (T cells are essentially devoid of these receptors, except for a small subset of T cells called Tγ cells.) These receptors, CD32 or FcγRII, have low affinity for the Fc portion of immunoglobulin and result in circulating B cells with loosely bound IgG and IgA on their surface in addition to the membrane-embedded IgM and IgD (Winchester *et al.,* 1975; Ammann *et al.,* 1977; Chao and Yokoyama, 1977; Ravetch and Kinet, 1991). The Fc receptors may be probed with labeled antibody–antigen aggregates that bind with high affinity to the receptors (Winchester and Ross, 1986). This information may be helpful in diagnosing cellular immune deficiencies or lymphoproliferative disorders.

The presence of B cells in a population of mononuclear cells often is detected using labeled anti-IgM antibody. (Macrophages and granulocytes have receptors for IgG, but not for IgM.) Lymphocytes incubated with labeled anti-IgM will bind the antibody by virtue of the IgM on their surface. If a fluorescent label is used, B cells may be identified by visual observation of the fluorescence by fluorescence microscopy or FACS. If an enzyme or colloid label is used, an opaque colored product is deposited around the cell and visualized by light microscopy.

Since lymphocytes have Ig receptors, the labeled anti-IgM also may bind to these receptors through their Fc portions. However, this occurs only if the anti-IgM complexes first with residual serum IgM not washed from the sample. These large complexes, but not free anti-IgM, bind well to the Ig receptors. To prevent this problem further, $F(ab')_2$ fragments of the anti-IgM, which have no Fc portion and cannot bind to cell-surface Ig receptors, may be used to probe the cell.

Experiment

In this experiment, cells with surface IgM will be detected in mouse spleen cells. Peroxidase- or colloidal gold-labeled anti-IgM will be incubated with smears of the cells. Any cells that bind the labeled antibody will be visualized with light microscopy. The peroxidase will deposit an insoluble intense brown product around the cell, distinguishing it from unlabeled neighbors. The gold label will be detected with silver deposited from an enhancement solution.

Spleen cells tend to give clearer staining than blood leukocytes. This may reflect the composition of the spleen cells, which contain at least 50% B cells whereas only 10–15% of peripheral blood lymphocytes are B cells.

IgM is visualized easily with readily available inexpensive antibodies. (Monoclonals to other surface antigens are quite expensive.) In addition, enzyme- or gold-labeled antibodies were chosen over fluorescent labeling to avoid a requirement for fluorescent microscopes.

Human peripherial blood leulocytes may also be stained by a similar procedure after isolating the cells by density centrifugation (Boyum 1968). However, the possibility of HIV- and hepatitis-infected blood precludes the use of human blood in the classroom laboratory unless extreme caution is used in handling and disposal of all blood-tainted materials. It is not recommended.

Materials

Materials common to enzymatic and gold labeling procedures

□ fixing solution (9.25% formaldehyde, 45% acetone in phosphate buffer)
    25 ml 37% formaldehyde
    45 ml acetone
    20 mg NaH_2PO_4
    100 mg KH_2PO_4

☐ tissue culture or balanced salt solution (e.g., Hank's, Dulbecco's; optional)

☐ PBS, pH 7.2 (0.15 M NaCl, 0.010 M potassium phosphate)

☐ bovine serum albumin (1% in PBS)

☐ Mayer's hematoxylin stain

☐ microscope slides

☐ desktop clinical centrifuge

☐ 15-ml plastic or glass clinical centrifuge tubes

☐ Petri dishes with moistened filter paper

☐ 37°C incubator

☐ stopcock grease and cotton-tipped applicator sticks

☐ 70% ethyl or isopropyl alcohol

☐ mice, any strain; immunized mice may present a greater number of IgM-positive cells

☐ scissors and forceps for removing spleen

☐ Petri dish

☐ bovine serum albumin (5% in PBS)

☐ 15-ml conical centrifuge tubes

☐ peroxidase-conjugated anti-mouse IgM (μ chain specific)

Antibody to mixed immunoglobulins IgA, IgG, and IgM also may be used, but specificity of cell labeling is lost. Further, biotin-labeled anti-IgM may be used, followed by enzyme or gold protein A.

☐ diaminobenzidene (DAB) substrate solution: 6 mg DAB in 10 ml 0.05 M Tris, 0.03% H_2O_2, pH 7.5.

Make immediately before use. CAUTION! DAB is a carcinogen and should be handled with gloves while wearing a mask.

Additional materials needed when using gold-labeled antibody

□ gold-conjugated anti-mouse IgM (µ chain specific)

□ silver enhancement solution (SilvEnhance LM, Zymed #49-0035)

Procedure

This experiment requires time on two separate days, but may be intermeshed with other procedures. Previous experience in handling cells and preparing slides is helpful, and may be acquired by preparing blood cell films, staining, and examining by light microscopy for leukocyte morphology.

Preparation of Cell Slides

DAY ONE

All operations are done at room temperature

1. Prepare in advance, a Petri dish with 5 ml PBS, pasture pipets, scissors, forceps, 70% alcohol, 15-ml centrifuge tubes.

2. Sacrifice a mouse by cervical dislocation or, preferably, asphyxiation in CO_2. Immediately wash the belly with alcohol, dab dry, and cut into the peritoneal cavity on the left side. Locate the spleen, a 1–2-cm long, flat, dark red organ and remove into a Petri dish containing 5 ml PBS.

3. Cut across the center of the spleen and tease the interior cells out into the buffer with the forceps and scissors. The spleen is a friable organ and should be disrupted easily.

4. Suction the cell suspension up and down several times with a pasteur pipet to break up any pieces of tissue, but be gentle; cells may be destroyed if handled too roughly. Transfer the suspension into a 15-ml conical centrifuge tube and allow large particulates to settle for 1–2 min. Remove the supernatant containing mostly single cells and transfer to another 15-ml centrifuge tube.

5. Centrifuge at 250–350 g for 5–10 min to pellet the cells. Wash the pellet twice with PBS or tissue culture medium. Wash by gentle suspension in

10 ml buffer followed by centrifugation. Resuspend the final pellet with 0.5 ml PBS containing 5% BSA. Keep on ice if not used immediately.

6. Clean 10 microscope slides with a brief dip in alcohol and wipe dry. Place one small drop, 50 µl, of cells onto the center of each slide and spread over a 2 × 2-cm area. Allow to dry in a horizontal position at room temperature for at least 1 hr and preferably overnight.

Immunostaining the Cells

DAY TWO

The procedure will be given for mouse splenocytes using peroxidase-labeled anti-mouse IgM. Gold-labeled antibody may be substituted for the peroxidase-labeled antibody, and the slides developed according to Step 7.

1. Fix the cells to the previously prepared dried slides by dipping a slide into fixing solution for 30 sec. Immediately after dipping, rinse the slide briefly in a beaker of distilled water and for 5 min in a beaker of PBS.

2. Flick the slide to remove drops of PBS and dry the bottom and the top of the slide with a Kimwipe, *except* for a 1-cm circle inside the cell area. Encircle this wet cell zone with a narrow band of stopcock grease applied with the tip of a cotton applicator stick. Do not apply a heavy band of grease; use just enough to retard the flow of liquid reagents added later (see margin note). Prepare four slides in this manner, keeping the cell area wet with PBS until antibody is added.

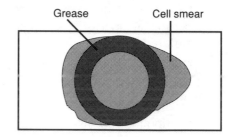

Grease   Cell smear

3. Prepare three dilutions of the peroxidase–anti-IgM that fall in the range suggested by the manufacturer. Try 1/100, 1/500, and 1/1000 for polyclonal antibodies; if monoclonal antibodies are used, a 1/20–1/500 dilution may be needed. Dilute the antibody in 1% BSA in PBS.

4. Gently apply 0.5 ml of each antibody dilution to separate slides, and 0.5 ml 1% BSA in PBS buffer to the fourth slide as a blank to test for endogenous peroxidase activity in the cells. Incubate for a minimum of 30 min at room

Volumes of 100–200 µl may be used if a small piece of parafilm is placed over the antibody to spread it over the cell smear.

temperature or overnight at 4°C. Lay the slides flat in a preferably air-tight or humidified atmosphere, for example, a wet filter paper-lined Petri dish, flat-bottomed plastic food storage container, or slide box.

5. Rinse the slide with PBS. Then place it in a Coplin jar or beaker of PBS for 5 min. Repeat once more with fresh PBS. At this point, the slides may be used immediately or air-dried after a quick rinse in water. If gold-labeled antibody is used, fix the slides again for 2 min in the formaldehyde/acetone solution, skip Step 6, and silver enhance according to Step 7.

6. Develop the peroxidase by applying 0.5 ml peroxidase substrate solution. During the development, view the slide under low power with a bright field microscope to evaluate the extent of staining. The DAB substrate develops rapidly to form an orange-brown precipitate around any labeled cells; care must be taken to stop development before background staining obscures positive cells. Stop development by rinsing the slide first in PBS, then in water, and finally air drying. Proceed to Step 8.

   Make sure all rinsing steps are gentle so that cells are not dislodged from the slide.

7. Gold-labeled antibodies are detected by applying a commercial silver enhancement solution. The development should be followed by low power bright field microscopy. The color develops over 15–30 min and progresses from a light pink to a brown-black. Do not keep the microscope light source on constantly during development, since the light may photoreduce the silver and cause increased background staining. Development should be stopped before individual cells are obscured. Stop development by rinsing 1–2 min in water and air drying. Proceed to Step 8.

8. Counterstain the slide with Mayer's hematoxylin or another nuclear stain, according to manufacturer's directions, with air drying and observe with bright field microscopy under oil immersion. Identify the lymphocytes and determine the percentage that is stained with peroxidase (or gold) label. This may be difficult for an untrained individual, especially if the fixing causes morphological changes in the cells. In this case, perhaps determining the distribution of *all* labeled cells in the total cell population would be more appropriate.

REFERENCES

Ammann, A. J., Borg, D., Kondo, L., and Wara, D. W. (1977). Quantitation of B cells in peripheral blood by polyacrylamide beads coated with anti-human chain antibody. *J. Immunol. Methods* **17,** 365–371.

Bierer, B. E., and Burakoff, S. J. (1988). T cell adhesion molecules. *FASEB J.* **2,** 2584–2590.

Boyum, A. (1968). Separation of leukocytes from blood and bone marrow. *Scan. J. Clin. Lab. Invest. (Suppl. 97)* **21,** 77.

Carter, R. H., and Fearon, D. T. (1992). CD19: Lowering the threshold for antigen receptor stimulation of B lymphocytes. *Science* **256,** 105–107.

Chao, W., and Yokoyama, M. M. (1977). Determination of B lymphocyte population using antibody-coated polyacrylamide beads. *Clin. Chim. Acta* **78,** 79–84.

Cordell, J. L., Falini, B., Erber, W. N., Ghosh, A. K., Abdulaziz, Z., MacDonald, S., Pulford, K. A. F., Stein, H., and Mason, D. Y. (1984). Immunoenzymatic labeling of monoclonal antibodies using immune complexes of alkaline phosphatase and monoclonal anti-alkaline phosphatase (APAAP complexes). *J. Histochem. Cytochem.* **32,** 219–229.

Danscher, G. and Norgaard, J. O. R. (1983). Light microscopic visualization of colloidal gold on resin-embedded tissue. *J. Histochem. Cytochem.* **31,** 1394–1398.

De Waele, M., Renmans, W., Segers, E., De Valck, V., and Jochmans, K. (1989). An immunogold-silver staining method for detection of cell surface antigens in cell smears. *J. Histochem. Cytochem.* **37,** 1855–1862.

Hsu, S. M., Raine, L., and Fanger, H. (1981). The use of avidin–biotin–peroxidase complex (ABC) in immunoperoxidase technique: A comparison between ABC and unlabeled antibody (PAP) procedures. *J. Histochem. Cytochem.* **29,** 577–580.

Jackson, A. L., and Warner, N. (1986). Preparation, staining, and analysis by flow cytometry of peripheral blood leukocytes. *In "Manual of Clinical Laboratory Immunology," 3d Ed.* (N. R. Rose, H. Friedman, and J. L. Fahey, eds.), pp. 226–235. American Society of Microbiology Press, Washington, D.C.

Klein, J. (1990). *In "Immunology,"* pp. 31–33. Blackwell Scientific Publications, Boston.

Knapp, W., Rieber, P., Dorken, B., Schmidt, R. E., Stein, H., and Kr.v.d.Borne, A. E. G. (1989). Towards a better definition of human leucocyte surface molecules. *Immunol. Today* 253–258.

Ravetch, J. V., and Kinet, J.-P. (1991). Fc receptors. *Annu. Rev. Immunol.* **9,** 457–492.

Shapiro, H. M. (1988). "Practical Flow Cytometry," 2d Ed. Wiley–Liss, New York.

Sternberger, L. A. (1978). "Immunocytochemistry." Prentice-Hall, Englewood Cliffs, New Jersey.

Strominger, J. (1989). Developmental biology of T cell receptors. *Science* **244,** 943–950

Winchester, R. J., and Ross, G. D. (1986). Methods for enumerating cell populations by surface markers with conventional microscopy. *In "Manual of Clinical Laboratory Immunology," 3d Ed.* (N. R. Rose, H. Friedman, and J. L. Fahey, eds.), pp. 212–225. American Society of Microbiology Press, Washington, D.C.

Winchester, R. J., Fu, S. M., Hoffman, T., and Kunkel, H. G. (1975). IgG on lymphocyte surfaces; technical problems and the significance of a third cell population. *J. Immunol.* **114,** 1210–1212.

Enzyme-Linked Immunosorbent Assay: ELISA

The ELISA, first introduced by Engvall and Perlman in 1971, has become the most popular immunoassay used in research laboratories today. The assay may be configured to measure antigens or antibodies with great sensitivity and specificity using relatively little equipment. Although other immunoassay formats exist, the ELISA provides three characteristics that often make it the format of choice. First, a solid-phase adsorbent allows quick and thorough washing of unbound reagents. The solid phase may consist of paper, plastic or glass beads, latex emulsions, or microtiter plate wells. Second, the enzyme label provides a safe, stable, and sensitive signal compared with another common label, the radionuclide. Finally, ELISAs are relatively trouble-free to develop, allowing even novices in the field to create an assay suitable for their needs. Indeed, because the ELISA has been the dominant immunoassay in the last decade, many researchers do not realize that other immunoassay formats exist. (For a review of other immunoassays, see Engvall, 1980; Nilsson, 1990; Parker, 1990).

This experiment will develop an antibody "sandwich" immunoassay suitable for detecting protein antigens. Although this assay is preferred for many antigens, additional assay formats for both antigen and antibody detection will be reviewed.

ELISAs for Antigen Detection

Antibody Sandwich Immunoassay

This assay may be the most versatile and sensitive for the detection of proteins of any ELISA: no purified antigen is required, only a suitable antibody. However, only multivalent antigens with different or repeating epitopes may be detected in this assay, since binding of two antibodies to the antigen is required. This requirement is normally not a limitation for proteins, which are almost always multivalent.

In this assay, a plastic microtiter plate is the solid phase on which the assay is performed. Microtiter plates have 96 wells, allowing 96 samples to be assayed under identical conditions. Each step in this assay will be described in more detail (Figure 10.1).

1. *Adsorption of antigen-specific primary antibody to a plastic well.* The antibody is noncovalently bound to the plastic by hydrophobic interactions. Although no covalent bonds are formed, the antibody remains bound during treatment with most detergents and moderate levels of pH and salt concentration. If an antibody adsorbs poorly to the plate, chemically modified plates are available that allow covalent attachment. After antibody adsorption, the well is blocked with a high concentration of a nonspecific protein: bovine serum albumin, gelatin, skim milk, or γ globulin.

2. *Addition of sample antigen with primary antibody.* Incubation times may be as short as 1 hr or as long as 1 day for maximum sensitivity. The incubation buffer often contains low concentrations of a nonionic detergent (Triton X-100 or Tween 20) and a carrier protein, which are included to reduce nonspecific adsorption of antigen to the plastic well.

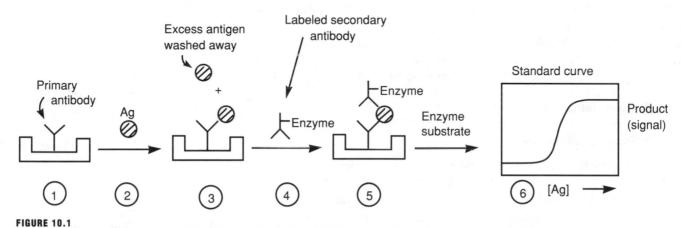

FIGURE 10.1

Antibody sandwich immunoassay. See text for description of Steps 1–6.

3. *Any antigen not bound to primary antibody is washed away.* Washing is facilitated by the well, which allows easy removal of wash buffer by suction or simple inversion. Thorough washing is essential to maintain a low background. This step, and most of the others, has been automated for high volume assays.

4. *Incubation of plate with enzyme-labeled second antibody.* The second antibody must bind antigen at an epitope different from that bound to the primary antibody. Thus, a single monoclonal cannot be used for both primary and second antibody (except if the epitope is repeated on the antigen), but two different monoclonals may be effective in the assay. However, a single polyclonal preparation may be used for both primary and second antibody, since the heterogeneous response normally includes antibodies against many different epitopes on one antigen. Affinity-purified polyclonal antibody works best, but an IgG fraction is often satisfactory.

   There are many variations on the type of second antibody used. For instance, the second antibody may be labeled with biotin and then detected by enzyme-labeled streptavidin, or an unlabeled second antibody may be detected with a third enzyme-labeled antibody specific for the isotype of the secondary antibody (see "Labeled Secondary Amplification Molecules").

5. *Labeled antibody binds to antigen bound by primary antibody.* Excess labeled antibody is washed away.

6. *Labeled antibody is detected by the addition of an enzyme substrate that is converted to a colored or fluorogenic product.* The product signal is plotted against antigen concentration to generate a standard curve.

Although this assay is one of the more sensitive enzyme immunoassays, it does require substantial amounts of both primary antibody and labeled second antibody. In addition, unless a purified source of the antigen is available as a standard, only relative, not absolute, amounts of antigen may be determined.

Antibody Capture Immunoassay

Although the sandwich assay may be the most sensitive immunoassay, the antibody capture assay requires fewer steps and is able to measure both low and high molecular weight antigens (Figure 10.2). In the capture assay, a preparation of antigen is adsorbed directly onto the microtiter well without the use of a primary antibody. Next, sample antigen along with labeled antibody is added to the well. Both adsorbed and sample antigen compete for the binding of the labeled antibody. Following an incubation period, the amount of antibody bound to adsorbed antigen is related inversely to the antigen concentration in the sample. Note that the standard curve is reversed from that of the sandwich assay.

A key problem in this assay is the coating of the plate with antigen. Substantial amounts of pure or partially pure antigen are required to coat the wells; for rare antigens, this is a difficult problem to surmount. In addition, some antigens may require covalent chemistries or intermediate binding molecules to be bound effectively (e.g., nucleic acids adsorb poorly to plastic and often are biotinylated and bound to streptavidin-coated plates, or bound to an amine plate with a phosphoramidite bond). Low molecular weight antigens, less that 1000 gm/mol, are called haptens and usually bind poorly to plastic. The haptens often are coupled covalently to a carrier protein; the carrier–hapten complex then is adsorbed to the

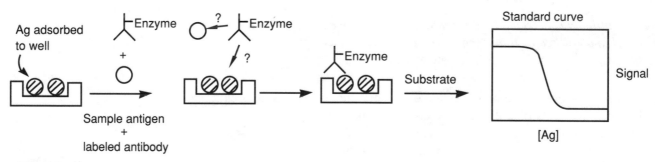

FIGURE 10.2

Antibody capture immunoassay.

plastic. However, some antigens are refractory to binding and may never be effective in this assay format.

One advantage is that labeled primary antibody is not required, since labeled secondary molecules may be used as the final signal (see "Labeled Secondary Amplification Molecules").

Antigen Capture Immunoassay

Although the sandwich and antibody capture assays are effective in measuring high molecular weight antigens, they may be less effective for low molecular weight antigens. The *antigen* capture assay measures low molecular weight antigens effectively by incorporating a labeled antigen. In this assay, a constant amount of *labeled* antigen is added to the *unlabeled* sample antigen. Both antigens then compete for binding to primary antibody on the plate. The greater the sample antigen concentration, the less labeled antigen is bound to antibody, and the smaller the final signal (Figure 10.3).

To increase the sensitivity of this assay, the sample antigen may be preincubated with the antibody, followed by a second incubation with the labeled antigen. Only radioactively or fluorescently labeled antigens are used in the assay. An enzyme-labeled antigen would be too large to allow effective antibody binding.

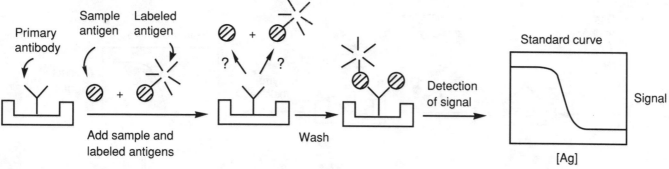

FIGURE 10.3

Antigen capture immunoasssay.

ELISA for Antibody Detection

Indirect Antibody Capture Immunoassay

The indirect antibody capture immunoassay (Figure 10.4) is used for detecting the presence of *antibody* rather than antigen in a test sample. It is used commonly to screen hybridoma fusions for antibody-producing cells or to screen antisera for antibody production. The assay requires fairly large quantities of pure or partially pure antigen to coat the plate, but uses commercially available labeled secondary antibody. First, the antibody sample is added to an antigen-coated well. If the sample contains antigen-specific antibody, the antibody binds to the well and is detected by a labeled isotype-specific secondary antibody. Thus, the "captured" test antibody is detected indirectly with a second labeled antibody.

Sensitivity and Reproducibility of ELISAs

Antibody sandwich assays usually are more sensitive than capture assays for detecting proteins, since they are capable of detecting as little as 0.1 ng/ml (pmol) antigen. However, antibody capture assays are preferred for low molecular weight antigens, typically measuring 1–10 pmol antigen, but having the potential to detect less.

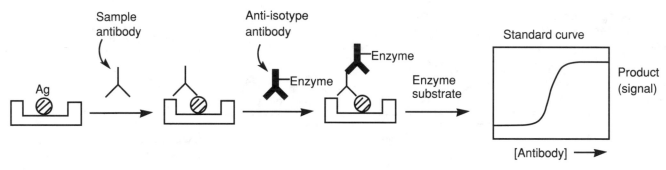

FIGURE 10.4

Indirect antibody capture immunoassay.

Several important parameters determine the ultimate sensitivity and reproducibility of an immunoassay. First, a high affinity antibody that binds an accessible epitope(s) is necessary for a sensitive assay. Second, the adsorption of antibody (or antigen) to the plate should not reduce the binding of antigen to antibody. The adsorption may orient the bound molecules in an ineffective manner or cause slight protein structure changes that lower or modify antibody binding. Fortunately, this does not appear to be a common problem; shifting to a different format often reduces any problems. Third, consistent incubation times, identical buffers and reagents, and redundant standard curves must be done for every plate to achieve reproducible results.

Enzyme Labels Used in ELISA

The two most popular labels for ELISA are alkaline phosphatase and horseradish peroxidase. Both enzymes have excellent stability, high turnover numbers, consistent conjugation, and a variety of substrates (see Experiment 6). However, each enzyme has its drawbacks. Peroxidase is inhibited by azide, which is used often as a preservative in biochemical buffers; it also has a smaller linear range in a dose–response curve than does alkaline phosphatase. Alkaline phosphatase has a poorly visible chromogenic substrate, p-nitrophenyl phosphate, and may occur as an endogenous enzyme in some biological samples. However, alkaline phosphatase has a fluorescent substrate, methyl umbelliferyl phosphate, that increases the sensitivity of phosphatase significantly, but requires an expensive fluorometer; thus, it normally is used only for high-volume sensitive assays. A new enzyme-coupled NADPH-containing substrate is claimed to be 10–100-fold more sensitive than p-nitrophenyl phosphate (ELISA Amplification System, Bethesda Research Laboratories).

Labeled Secondary Amplification Molecules

All ELISAs require an enzyme to produce the final signal. Although the primary antibody may be labeled, many ELISAs use labeled *secondary* molecules (Figure 10.5). For instance, enzyme-labeled isotype-specific antibody or enzyme-labeled protein A may be used to detect primary antibody. Alternatively, biotin-labeled secondary antibody or biotin–protein A may bind to primary antibody, fol-

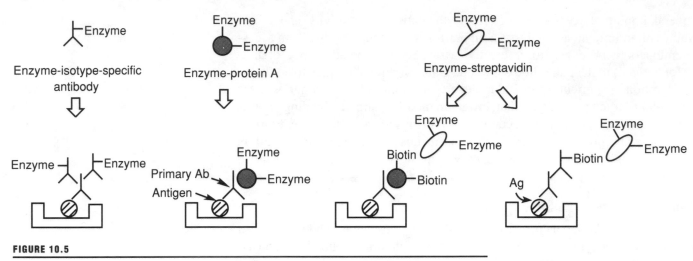

FIGURE 10.5

Secondary amplification systems.

lowed by enzyme-labeled streptavidin. These indirect systems often amplify the original antibody–antigen interaction by building up layers of molecules that increase the final signal. However, every added layer also increases the possibility of nonspecific binding and higher background signal!

Experiment

In this experiment, a sandwich assay for glucose oxidase will be developed using the biotin- and the peroxidase-labeled anti-glucose oxidase antibodies prepared in Experiment 7. For greatest sensitivity combined with lowest background, the primary antibody and the secondary antibody will be titrated for optimal concentrations. A more complete optimization would vary buffers, incubation times, incubation temperatures, and enzyme labels.

Materials

□ affinity-purified anti-glucose oxidase (Experiment 5)

□ HRP- or alkaline phosphatase-labeled anti-glucose oxidase (Experiment 6)

□ biotin-labeled anti-glucose oxidase (Experiment 6)

□ HRP or alkaline phosphatase streptavidin [e.g., Zymed Laboratories, #43-4323 (HRP); #43-4322 (alkaline phosphatase)]

□ glucose oxidase, 0.7–500 ng/ml in TBT

□ 0.10 M sodium carbonate buffer, pH 9.5

□ TBS (Appendix B)

□ TBS with 1% bovine serum albumin

□ TBT (TBS with 0.1% BSA and 0.01% Triton X-100)

□ HRP substrate solutions [prepare either *o*-phenylenediamine (OPD) or 2,2′-azinodi(3-ethylbenzothiazoline-6-sulfonic acid) (ATBS) substrate *just before use*]

OPD (read at 405, 416, or 490 nm)
30 mg *o*-phenylenediaminedihydrochloride
3 ml 1 M citrate, pH 4.7
27 ml water
125 μl 3% H_2O_2

ATBS (read at 405 or 416 nm)
15 mg 2,2′-azinodi(3-ethylbenzothiazoline-6-sulfonic acid), diammonium salt
3 ml 1 M citrate, pH 4.7
27 ml water
300 μl 3% H_2O_2

☐ alkaline phosphatase substrate solution (prepare *just before use*)
   PNPP (read at 405 nm)
      30 mg *p*-nitrophenyl phosphate, ammonium salt
      3 ml 0.5 M $NaCO_3$, pH 9.5
      24 ml water
      3 ml 0.005 M $MgCl_2$

☐ 96 well microtiter plates (Immulon 2 or 4, Dynatech # 011-010-3450 or # 011-010-3850, Nunc Immuno Plate "Maxisorp" F96, # 439454)

☐ 8 or 12 needle manifold for aspirating reagents from microtiter plates (optional)

☐ 12-channel micropipet, 25–250 µl capacity (optional) (Flow Multichannel Pipette, # 77-705-00)

☐ microtiter plate reader (optional, but highly desirable) (Flow Titertek Multi-scan MCC/340, # 78-626-00)

☐ 500-ml plastic squeeze wash bottles to hold TBT buffer for washing steps

Procedure

This procedure uses HRP- or alkaline phosphatase-labeled anti-glucose oxidase as the secondary sandwich antibody. If biotin-labeled antibody is used, an additional step is necessary, given as Step 10b, which extends the assay by 1 day.

Never allow the plate to dry out between steps. If you must wait, fill the plate with TBT, cover, and store at 4°C until the next step is performed.

Step 1: Coat the microtiter plate with three different concentrations of primary antibody

DAY ONE

1. Identify plate with an indelible marker on top and sides.

2. Prepare three 10-ml dilutions of affinity purified anti-glucose oxidase in 0.10 M sodium carbonate buffer, pH 9.5. Although this buffer concentration and pH are used frequently, a complete optimization procedure would investigate variations in both of these parameters. The dilutions to prepare are

The time of incubations may vary considerably. Six- to 24-hr incubation times are often required for adequate binding at 4°C, while 1–2 hr at room temperature or 30–60 minutes at 37°C is often sufficient. The protocol below is extended to allow time for short (3 hr) lab sections, prelab lectures, and preparation of dilutions for selected reagents. However, after an ELISA is optimized, it may be routinely completed in 1 day.

The affinity purified anti-glucose oxidase will be used to coat the plastic wells. To investigate the effect of antibody purity, students could coat plates with the γ-globulin fraction obtained in Experiment 3. Further, the coating buffer pH could be varied (pH 7, 0.10 M phosphate; pH 8, 0.05 M borate) to investigate pH influence on antibody binding.

(a) 10 ml 0.10 µg/ml anti-glucose oxidase

(b) 10 ml 1.0 µg/ml anti-glucose oxidase

(c) 10 ml 10 µg/ml anti-glucose oxidase

3. Aliquot 200 µl of each dilution into the rows of the plate as pictured in Figure 10.6.

   Seal with a transparent tape cover or parafilm. Set in refrigerator at 4°C to incubate 24–48 hr. Incubation for 2–4 hr at room temperature is also successful. To avoid splashing samples within the wells, be careful not to tip or jar the plate sharply.

Primary antibody concentrations greater than 10 µg/ml do not increase the amount adsorbed to the plate.

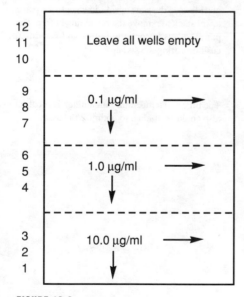

FIGURE 10.6

Prepared microtiter plate.

Step 2: Coat the plate with blocking protein

DAY TWO

4. Suction fluid off all wells. This can be done quickly with a pasteur pipet or an 8-needle manifold attached with rubber tubing to a vacuum flask. Again, avoid sharp jarring of the plate.

5. Immediately flood each well (fill to the top) with 1% BSA in TBS. Use a wash bottle filled with the buffer and gently squirt into the wells in an even motion, avoiding large bubbles in the wells. Incubate 30 min at room temperature or store at 4°C for 24 hr. Coat all wells, including rows 10–12.

6. "Whap out" 1% BSA in TBS and wash plate three times (3×) with TBT. For each washing, hold the empty plate over a sink and squirt buffer from a wash bottle into the empty wells. Flood the wells with buffer, avoiding large bubbles in the wells since this decreases effective washing. Extra buffer will drip into the sink. Allow 2–3 min for molecules to desorb from the wells; then whap out the wash buffer. After the last wash, fill the plate with buffer and proceed to Step 7 or cover and store at 4°C.

The plate is now coated with primary antibody.

Step 3: Incubate glucose oxidase antigen in the antibody-coated plate

7. Prepare serial 3-fold dilutions of glucose oxidase in TBT as shown in Table 10.1. (Prepare 4 ml of each dilution.)

8. Empty the plate. (Whap out.) Add 200 µl of each glucose oxidase sample to the wells, according to row letter (A–G, Step 7; see Figure 10.7). Add buffer to all wells in row H as blank controls. Incubate 18–24 hr at 4°C, or 4–6 hr at room temperature.

DAY THREE

9. Empty the plate by suction; then wash the plate four times with TBT.

Some investigators note that storing an antibody (or antigen)-coated plate in the presence of a high concentration of blocking protein (BSA) for extended periods of time may reduce the amount of antibody bound. This presumably occurs because the blocking protein competes the antibody off the plastic. If antibody-coated plates are not to be used within 2–3 days, it may be best to keep the original coating antibody solutions in the plate during the storage period and block with protein immediately before use.

"Whap out" wash buffers as follows. Next to a sink, place a stack of paper towels about 0.5 cm thick. Take the microtiter plate, quickly invert, and snap the buffer out into the sink, shaking several times to dislodge most of the fluid. Then, quickly snap the plate upside down onto the paper towel stack to remove the remaining buffer. The paper towels absorb the buffer and provide a cushion during the "whap!"

The time and temperature for antigen incubation also could be studied to optimize the assay.

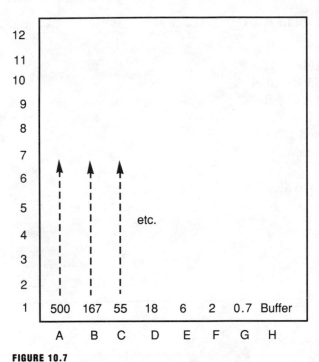

FIGURE 10.7

Prepared microtiter plate with glucose oxidase.

TABLE 10.1

Distribution of Glucose Oxidase in Microtiter Plate

Glucose oxidase (ng/ml)	Row number
500	A
167	B
55	C
18	D
6	E
2	F
0.7	G

Step 4: Add the labeled second antibody

If *enzyme-labeled* anti-glucose oxidase is used, go to Step 10a. If *biotin-labeled* anti-glucose oxidase is used, go to Step 10b. After either Step, continue to Step 11.

10a. Prepare three-10 ml dilutions of enzyme-labeled anti-glucose oxidase. The three dilutions should be 1/200, 1/800, and 1/3200 in TBT. Add 200 µl of the dilutions to the wells as shown in Figure 10.8. Incubate 18–24 hr at 4°C or 4–6 hr at room temperature. Go to Step 11.

10b. Prepare three 10-ml dilutions of biotin-labeled anti-glucose oxidase. The three dilutions should be 1/200, 1/800, and 1/3200 in TBT. Add 200 µl of the dilutions to the wells as shown in Figure 10.8. Incubate 18–24 hr at 4°C or 4–6 hr at room temperature. Wash plate four times with TBT. Add 200 µl HRP-streptavidin or alkaline phosphatase–streptavidin diluted 1/4000 in TBT. (The exact dilution will vary depending on the source, but usually 1/1000–1/4000 is a working dilution.)

Incubate 18–24 hr at 4°C or 2–4 hr at room temperature. Go to Step 11.

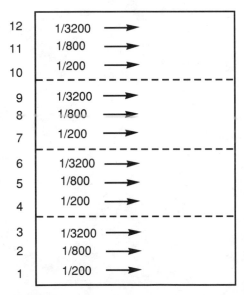

FIGURE 10.8

Prepared microtiter plate with anti-glucose oxidase.

DAY FOUR

11. Wash plate four times with TBT.

Step 5: Develop the plate to produce colored product

12. Develop the plate by adding the appropriate enzyme substrate solution (see *Materials*). Add 200 µl substrate solution to each well using a 12-channel micropipet for convenience (see instructor).

13. Read the plates on a microtiter plate reader at the appropriate wavelength after 10–30 min or when the blank wells (row H) are still colorless, but the sample wells show a satisfactory distribution of color. The blank plate pattern below may be used to record absorption data from each well for easy reference.

If the plate cannot be read immediately after development, quench by adding 25 µl 4 N H_2SO_4 to each well. Again, use the 12-channel pipet. For PNPP, do not quench with H_2SO_4 since this will protonate the yellow nitrophenol product and turn it colorless.

If a microtiter plate reader is not available, dilute 100 µl of each well into 3 ml 0.40 N H_2SO_4 (OPD) or 0.5 M carbonate, pH 9.5 (PNPP). Read each tube in a conventional spectrophotometer.

	1	2	3	4	5	6	7	8	9	10	11	12
A												
B												
C												
D												
E												
F												
G												
H												

14. Plot absorbance against glucose oxidase concentration (ng/ml) on semilog paper as shown in Figure 10.9.

Questions

1. How does the concentration of primary antibody affect the curve? Consider the background readings and the sensitivity of the curve.

2. How does the concentration of labeled second antibody affect the curve?

3. Which antibody, primary or secondary, influences the signal-to-noise ratio most? Can you tell?

4. Which part of the semilog plot is most sensitive to changes in antigen concentration: lower, middle, or upper?

5. How do the data look using a *linear* scale to plot glucose oxidase concentration?

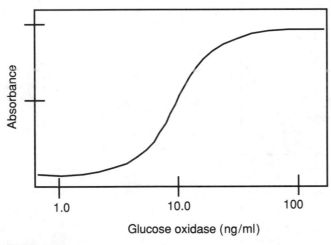

FIGURE 10.9

Plot of absorbance against glucose oxidase concentration.

REFERENCES

Engvall, E. (1980). Enzyme immunoassay ELISA and EMIT. *Meth. Enzymol.* **70**, 419–439.

Engvall, E., and Perlman, P. (1971). Enzyme-linked immunosorbent assay (ELISA): Quantitative assay of immunoglobulin G. *Immunochemistry* **8**, 871–879.

Nilsson, B. (1990). Enzyme-linked immunosorbent assays. *Curr. Opin. Immunol.* **2**, 898–904.

Parker, C. W. (1990). Immunoassays. *Meth. Enzymol.* **182**, 700–718.

Chemistries and Procedures for Affinity Chromatography

CHEMISTRIES FOR ACTIVATING SOLID PHASE SUPPORTS

Activating Agents

Chemical structures for some of these agents are shown in Figure 1.

CNBr Cyanogen bromide, used to activate polysaccharides such as agarose to a cyanate ester.

CDI   Carbodiimide. A water soluble version, EDC [1-ethyl-3-(3-dimethyl-aminopropyl) carbodiimide], is employed often in aqueous situations. This reagent couples amino to carbonyl groups, forming a peptide bond.

OXI   1,4-butanediol diglycidylether. This reagent activates hydroxyl groups on polysaccharides to reactive oxirane groups that bind amine- and hydroxyl-containing ligands.

CDM Carbonyldiimidazole. This reagent activates hydroxyl groups on polysac- charides to form an imidazole carbamate that reacts with amine-containing ligands.

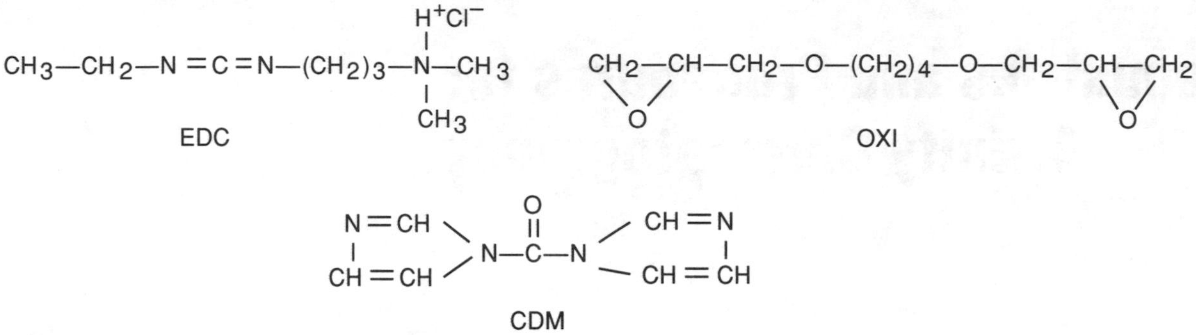

$$CH_3-CH_2-N=C=N-(CH_2)_3-\overset{\overset{\displaystyle H^+Cl^-}{|}}{\underset{\underset{\displaystyle CH_3}{|}}{N}}-CH_3$$

EDC

$$CH_2-CH-CH_2-O-(CH_2)_4-O-CH_2-CH-CH_2$$

OXI

$$\underset{CH=CH}{\overset{N=CH}{}}\!\!\!\diagdown N-\overset{\overset{\displaystyle O}{\|}}{C}-N\diagdown\!\!\!\underset{CH=CH}{\overset{CH=N}{}}$$

CDM

FIGURE 1

Some activating agents.

Agarose Activation

Agarose may be activated with CNBr, CDM, or OXI (Figure 2A–C) to bind amino ligands, NH$_2$–**R**, directly. Agarose also may be coupled with a diamine and treated with CDI to couple a carboxyl ligand, COOH–**R** ((Figure 2D). Finally, the heterobifunctional compound succinimidyl 3-(2-pyridyldithio)propionate (SPDP) often is employed to bind sulfhydryl-containing ligands, SH–**R**, to amino agarose (Figure 2E).

Polyacrylamide Activation

Polyacrylamide activation may occur by a displacement reaction with a base or directly with gluteraldehyde. These activation procedures result in a resin that may bind aldehyde (CHO–**R**; Figure 3A), amino (NH$_2$–**R**; Figure 3B), or carboxyl (COOH–**R**; Figure 3C) containing ligands.

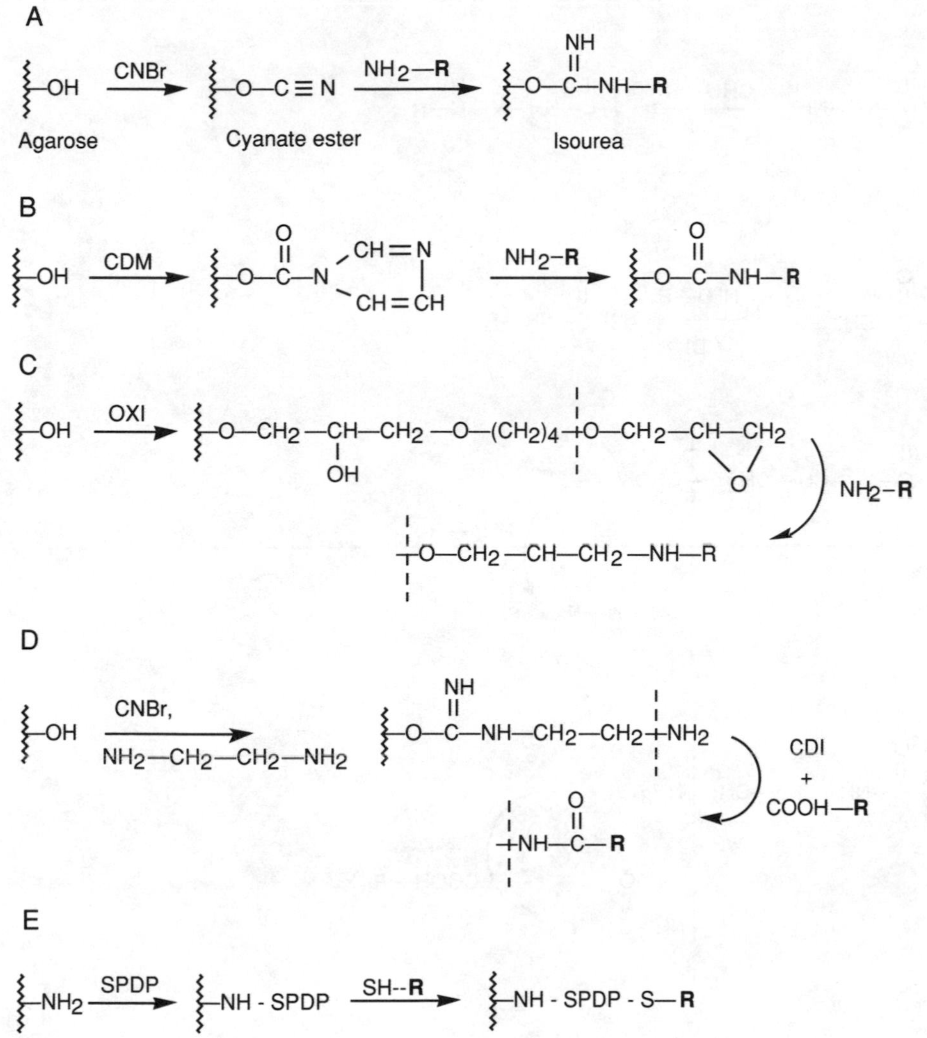

A

B

C

D

E

FIGURE 2

Agarose activation.

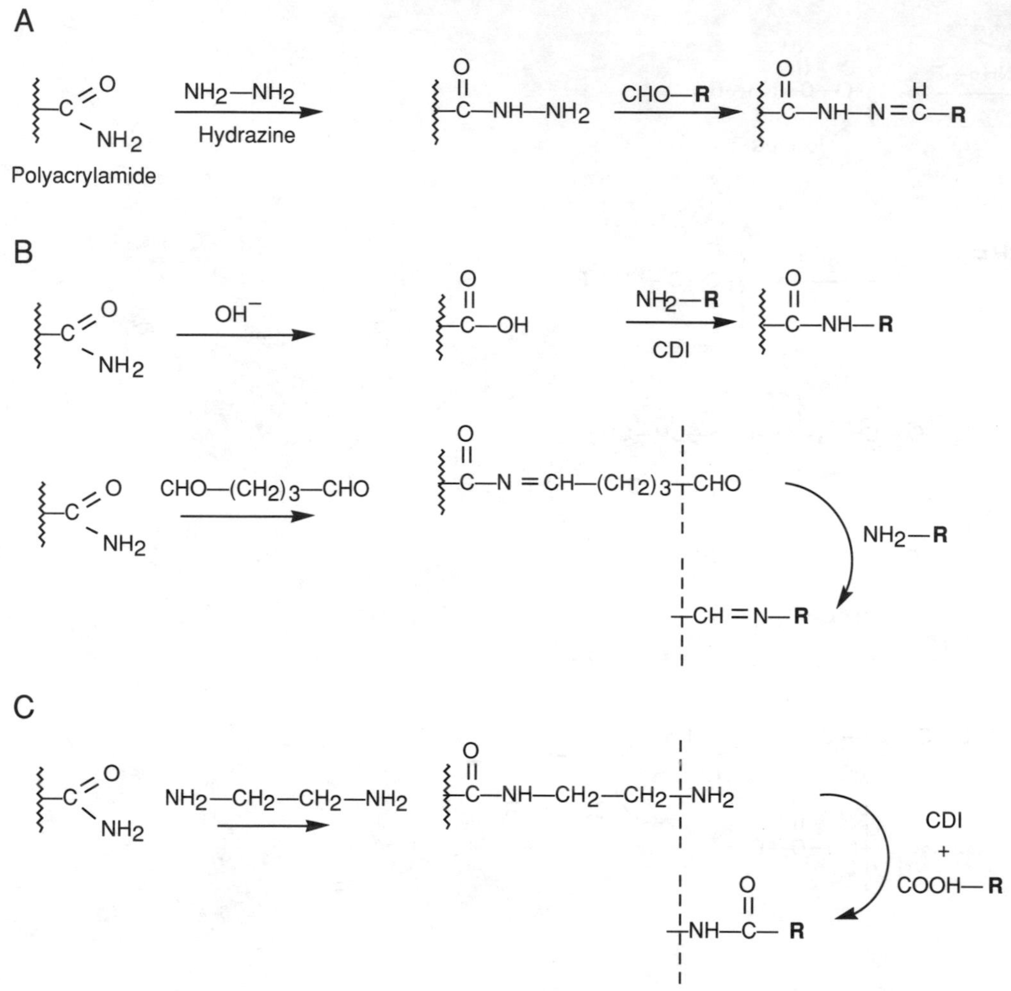

A

Polyacrylamide

B

C

FIGURE 3

Polyacrylamide activation.

140

PROCEDURES FOR CNBR-ACTIVATED AGAROSE

Method A. Using K_2CO_3 as Base

This procedure (March, Parikh, and Cuatrecasas, 1974) is the easiest, but results in a minimally activated gel. However, it is suitable for most large molecular weight protein ligands, when relatively few molecules of ligand are bound.

Materials

□ 50 ml packed moist agarose gel (Sepharose 4B or Sepharose CL-4B)

□ 2 M K_2CO_3, ice cold

□ 0.1 M $KHCO_3$, pH 9.0–9.2, ice cold

□ water, ice cold

□ 0.001 M HCl, ice cold

□ 5 gm CNBr, approximately 1 gm/ml in acetonitrile
    Weigh the solid CNBr in a tared sealed bottle, then add acetonitrile to dissolve, or purchase 5 M CNBr in acetonitrile (Aldrich # 26,161-0).

□ 0.5–10 mg/ml protein or 1–100 mM ligand in 0.1 M $KHCO_3$, pH 9.

□ fume hood

□ scintered glass funnel, coarse mesh (60 cm)

□ magnetic stir plate, stir bar

□ 2-liter filter flask

Procedure

Perform all operations with CNBr in the fume hood. All CNBr containing solutions are flushed down the fume hood drain with water for 5 to 10 min. **Wear gloves!** After the procedure, let all glassware dissipate CNBr in the fume hood overnight before cleanup.

1. Wash the agarose in water 2–3 times in a scintered glass funnel. After the last wash, suction to a moist gel. Transfer to a beaker with a capacity at least 4 times the gel volume.

2. Add 50 ml water and 50 ml 2 M KCO_3 to the agarose and cool in an ice bath with stirring.

3. Add 5 gm CNBr in acetonitrile (or 10 ml 5 M CNBr) to the stirring agarose. Allow to react for exactly 2 min.

4. Immediately filter through the scintered glass funnel and wash twice with ice cold water, then at least four times with 0.001 M HCl. After the last wash, leave the gel dry.

5. To the agarose, add the protein or ligand in 0.1 M $KHCO_3$, pH 9, and shake gently for approximately 12 hr at 4°C. Add enough volume of the ligand solution or of extra buffer to maintain a slurry that can be kept in suspension with gentle shaking. Stir bars are to be avoided to prevent breaking of the agarose beads.

6. After 12 hr, add 1 ml aminoethanol to the mixture to quench any unused cyanate ester groups on the gel. Allow to react at least 2 hr.

7. Wash the agarose, saving the first eluate to determine the amount of protein not bound to the agarose. A suggested series of washes includes

   0.1 M $KHCO_3$, pH 9.0–9.2

   1 M NaCl

   1 M NaCl , 0.1 M acetate, pH 4.5

   0.15 M NaCl, 0.01 M phosphate, pH 7.4

8. Store gel at 4°C. Add thimerosal or a few drops of chloroform as a bacteriostatic agent.

Method B. Using NaOH as Base

This procedure (Axen, Porath, and Ernback, 1967) requires more effort during the activation procedure, but results in an optimally activated gel suitable for low molecular weight and protein ligands.

Materials
- ☐ 50 ml packed moist agarose gel (Sepharose 4B or Sepharose CL-4B)
- ☐ 5 gm CNBr in acetonitrile (see *Materials*, Method A)
- ☐ 5 M NaOH
- ☐ water, ice cold
- ☐ 0.001 M HCl, ice cold
- ☐ 0.1 M KCO_3, pH 9.0–9.2, ice cold
- ☐ pH meter or pH paper
- ☐ fume hood
- ☐ magnetic stir plate, stir bar
- ☐ 2-liter filter flask
- ☐ scintered glass funnel, coarse mesh

Procedure
1. Stir 50 ml agarose into 50 ml water at 20°C.
2. Add 5 gm CNBr to the stirred agarose. Add 5 M NaOH to maintain the pH between 10 and 11. A pH meter or pH paper may be used with equivalent results.
3. Maintain the high pH for 10–15 min, being careful to maintain the temperature between 18 and 20°C by the addition of ice directly to the stirred mixture. Do not allow to rise above 22°C.
4. Immediately wash twice with ice cold water, then six times with 0.001 M HCl.

5. Add ligand or protein as in Step 5, Method A. Continue procedure according to Method A.

REFERENCES

Axen, R., Porath, J., and Ernback, S. (1967). Chemical coupling of peptides and proteins to polysaccharides by means of cyanogen halides. *Nature (London)* **214**, 1302–1304.

Inman, J. K. (1974). Covalent linkage of functional groups, ligands, and proteins to polyacrylamide beads. *Meth. Enzymol.* **34**, 30–58.

March, S. C., Parikh, I., and Cuatrecasas, P. (1974). A simplified method for cyanogen bromide activation of agarose for affinity chromatography. *Anal. Biochem.* **60**, 149–152.

Mosbach, R., Koch-Schmidt, A., and Mosbach, K. (1976). Immobilization of enzymes to various acrylic copolymers. *Meth. Enzymol.* **44**, 53–65.

Porath, J. (1974). General methods and coupling procedures. *Meth. Enzymol.* **34**, 13–30.

Kohn, J., and Wilchek, M. (1984). The use of cyanogen bromide and other novel cyamylating agents for the activation of polysaccharide resins. *Appl. Biochem. Biotechnol.* **9**, 285–304.

Schnaar, R. L., and Lee, Y. C. (1975). Polyacrylamide gels copolymerized with active esters. A new medium for affinity systems. *Biochemistry* **14**, 1535–1541.

Sundberg, L., and Porath, J. (1974). Attachment of group-containing ligands to insoluble polymers by means of bifunctional oxiranes. *J. Chromatography* **90**, 87–98.

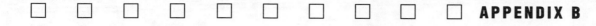

Buffers

Stoll and Blanchard (1990) provide an excellent review of buffers.

TBS

Tris Buffered Saline
(0.01 M Tris, 0.15 M NaCl, pH 7.4)
The buffering capacity of Tris (pKa = 8.3) at pH 7.4 is minimal compared with
phosphate (pKa = 7.2). Use PBS when possible at neutral pH.
    10X TBS stock (1 liter)
        87 gm NaCl
        12.1 gm Tris base [N-tris(hydroxymethyl)amino-methane, $(HOCH_3)CNH_3^+$]
        H_2O up to 1 liter
Adjust pH to 7.2 with 6 N HCl. Store at 4°C. Dilute 1 part 10X stock with 9 parts
water to use. Check pH of diluted stock; it should be 7.2–7.5.

TBT

Tris Buffered Saline with BSA and Triton X-100
(0.01 M Tris, 0.15 M NaCl, 1 mg/ml BSA, 0.01% Triton X-100, pH 7.4)
    TBS
    5 % w/v BSA (Dissolve 5.0 gm BSA in 100 ml water. Adjust to pH 7. Store
    frozen at –20°C.)
Add 20 ml 5% w/v BSA and 0.1 ml Triton X-100 per liter of TBS.

PBS

Phosphate Buffered Saline
(0.01 M phosphate, 0.15 M NaCl, pH 7.4)
    10X PBS stock (1 liter)
        87 gm NaCl
        18.2 gm K_2HPO_4-$3H_2O$
        2.3 gm KH_2PO_4
        H_2O up to 1 liter
Dilute 1 part stock with 9 parts water to use. Check pH of dilution; it should be
7.2–7.5

EDTA

Ethylene Diamine Tetraacetic Acid
(0.10 M EDTA, pH 7.4)
This is a stock solution that may be diluted with other buffer ingredients to obtain
the desired EDTA concentration.
    37.2 gm disodium EDTA
Dissolve in approximately 900 ml water. Adjust pH to 7.4 with 6 M NaOH, then
bring the total volume to 1 liter. EDTA is minimally soluble in water at neutral
pH. Molarities above 0.1 M do not stay in solution at refrigerator temperatures.

REFERENCE

Stoll, V. S., and Blanchard, J. S. (1990). Buffers: Principles and practice. *Meth.
    Enzymol.* **182,** 24–37.

PAGE Reagent and Staining Procedures

Experiments 7 and 8 require electrophoresis of protein samples on slab gels. To perform this electrophoresis, it is necessary to use slab gel electrophoresis apparatuses and power supplies and follow instructions provided by the equipment manufacturers to assemble the sandwich for the slab, cast gels, connect power supply to slab gel apparatus, and apply current. Recipes for typical-size slab gels are given below; volumes can be adjusted to accommodate other size slabs. While the recipes below are for SDS-PAGE if used as written, omitting SDS and mercapoethanol yields native gels.

STOCK SOLUTIONS FOR SDS STACKING GELS

Acrylamide: *bis* acrylamide
(30% T, 2.67% C)

29.2 gm acrylamide
0.8 gm N',N'-bis methylene acrylamide
Bring up to 100 ml with distilled water. Store at 4°C in an amber bottle up to 6 months

1.5 m Tris-Cl, pH 8.8

18.15 gm Tris base
80 ml distilled water
Adjust to pH 8.8 with 6 N HCl. Bring up to 100 ml with distilled water. Store at 4°C up to 6 months

0.5 m Tris-Cl, pH 6.8

3.0 gm Tris base

40 ml distilled water

Adjust to pH 6.8 with 6 N HCl. Bring up to 50 ml with distilled water. Store at 4°C up to 6 months

10% SDS (w/v)

10 gm sodium dodecyl sulfate

Bring up to 100 ml with distilled water. Store at room temperature.

Running Buffer, 4X Stock
(0.025 m Tris, 0.192 m glycine, 0.1% SDS, pH 8.3)

12.0 gm Tris base

57.6 gm glycine

4.0 gm SDS

Bring up to 1 liter with distilled water. Store at 4°C. Dilute with 3 parts water for use. Reuse buffer in lower chamber (anode) 4–5 times, but discard upper buffer after each run.

Sample Preparation Buffer (SPB) 4X Stock

1.0 ml Tris buffer, pH 6.8 (Solution C)

1.6 ml 10% SDS (Solution D)

0.8 ml glycerol

0.4 ml mercaptoethanol (or 23 mg dithiothreitol)

4.0 ml water

several crystals of bromophenol blue or *m*-cresol purple.

FOR USE: First, adjust the protein samples to approximately 0.5 mg/ml. Then add 1 part of the SPB to 3 parts protein sample, and heat at 95°C (boiling water) for 5–10 min or at 37°C for 30–60 min. Cool to room temperature before layering on gel. This concentration will allow application of 5 µg protein in a volume of 13 µl to the gel, an amount that will stain strongly with Coomassie Blue. Protein solutions to be treated with SPB should not contain more than 0.5 M salts for best results. Otherwise, precipitation of SDS and the sample proteins may occur.

Meta-cresol purple migrates ahead of small peptides, whereas bromophenol blue runs slightly behind. Store frozen at −20°C. May be rethawed many times.

NOTE: This is a reducing buffer; it will break all disulfide bonds. A nonreducing buffer may also be prepared by omitting the mercaptoethanol and adding additional water.

CASTING THE GELS

Gels normally are cast immediately after mixing the various components listed here. However, if all components except ammonium persulfate are mixed, the mixture will not polymerize and may be stored for 4–6 wk at 4°C. To initiate polymerization, add the final component, ammonium persulfate, and cast the gels according to manufacturer's instructions. Separating gels that have been cast also may be stored between their glass plates for several weeks at 4°C if tightly wrapped in plastic wrap. To use, place the gels in the casting apparatus and pour the stacking gel.

Separating Gel Preparation

40 ml are needed for two 14-cm × 14-cm × 0.75-mm slabs

10 ml are needed for two 8-cm × 5-cm × 0.75-mm slabs

Many procedures request that, prior to TEMED addition, the gel solution be deaerated for 10 min on a water aspirator to reduce variations in the gel during polymerization. This procedure normally is not needed, but may become necessary if slow or incomplete polymerization occurs. Different percentage gels separate different molecular weight ranges:

7.5% gels are useful for 25–200-kD proteins

10% gels are useful for 25–100-kD proteins

12% gels are useful for 10–100-kD proteins

| | Gel percentage | | | |
Reagent added in order listed	7.5	10	12	Volume measure
Distilled water	4.8	4.0	3.3	ml
1.5 M Tris-Cl, pH 8.8, Solution B	2.5	2.5	2.5	ml
10% (w/v) SDS	0.1	0.1	0.1	ml
Acrylamide: bis (30% T, 2.67% C)	2.5	3.3	4.0	ml
TEMED	5	5	5	μl
10% ammonium persulfate (fresh weekly) (to start polymerization)	25	25	25	μl
Total volume	10	10	10	ml

Mix by swirling and immediately pipet into gel plate sandwich. Overlay carefully with water or with water saturated *n*-butanol. Allow to polymerize at least 20 min or until a small sample of gel in a test tube hardens. The gel may be stored for a few weeks in the casting stand if the butanol or water is replaced by a 1/4 dilution of Solution B. The top of the gels should be wrapped tightly with plastic wrap to reduce drying during storage.

Stacking Gel Preparation
(4.0% gel, 0.125 m Tris, pH 6.8)

3.1 ml	distilled water
1.25 ml	0.5 m Tris-Cl, pH 6.8, Solution C
0.05 ml	10% (w/v) SDS
0.65 ml	acrylamide:bis (30% T, 2.67% C)
25 µl	10% ammonium persulfate (fresh)
2.5 ml	TEMED

The total volume should be 5 ml. Pour off the overlay solution from the polymerized separating gel, blot briefly with a paper wipe, and fill the gel plates to the top with the stacking gel solution. Quickly insert the comb, dislodging any small bubbles stuck at the bottom of the comb, and allow to polymerize at least 20 min or until a sample of gel solution in a test tube hardens. Gently remove the comb and place the gel in the electrophoresis unit. Cover with running buffer. You are now ready to apply samples to the gel.

APPLYING THE SAMPLES AND RUNNING THE GEL

Apply the Samples

After preparation of the samples with SPB, the sample should be applied after the gel has been placed in the electrophoresis tank and both the lower and the upper running buffer chambers have been filled. Apply the sample to a well with a Hamilton syringe or automatic micropipet. The volume applied should be kept to a minimum, usually 5–20 μl for a minigel and 20–100 μl for a standard gel. Ultimately, the volume of the well determines the maximum volume that may be applied.

The glycerol in the sample mixture will insure that the applied sample sinks to the bottom of the well.

Electrophorese the Samples

Electrophorese the gels at 70–100 V, 10–20 mA. To save time, try 150–200 V, but be sure to cool the gel adequately or the samples will migrate near the edges of the gel slower than samples near the center, creating smile-shaped pattern. The time for a minigel should be 60–90 min. Stop the run when the *m*-cresol purple runs off the bottom of the gel.

STAINING THE GELS

The gels may be stained with a variety of stains, the most common of which are presented in this section. The staining procedures presented in this section include protein stains (Coomassie staining, sensitive to 1–10 μg protein, and silver staining, sensitive to 10–100 μg protein) and carbohydrate stains, which are used to stain the carbohydrate on glycoproteins (fluorescent periodate staining, sensitive to 10–100 μg glycoprotein, and Con A–peroxidase staining, sensitive to 1–10 μg glycoprotein). Additional staining methods are included in the reference section.

Coomassie Stain for Protein

There are many variations on this stain recipe. Concentrations of Coomassie blue range from 0.025% to 0.5%, and all work reasonably well. Stains with high dye concentrations tend to give higher background color, but stain more quickly. Methanol concentrations also vary up to 40%, but this high concentration does not seem to be necessary, and is more costly. Finally, the acetic acid content should be at least 7% to maintain the protein in an insoluble state that will not diffuse from the gel and to keep the Coomassie dye in an anion form that will bind to the positive charges on the protein effectively. Coomassie G-250 gives better staining at a lower concentration of dye, but is more expensive.

Reagents

Stain

> 1 gm Coomassie brilliant blue R-250
> 200 ml methanol
> 100 ml glacial acetic acid

Dissolve dye in solvents, then bring up to 1 liter total volume with water. Filter the solution through #1 filter paper. Store at room temperature in amber bottles. Reuse many times until protein bands do not stain strongly.

Destain

> 100 ml methanol
> 70 ml acetic acid
> 530 ml water

Procedure

1. Cover the gels with 1 cm stain and shake gently for 1–16 hr at room temperature. Shaking is not necessary, but reduces stain time.

2. Destain by repeated 1–2 hr washings with destain. Preheating the destain or heating the gel while in destaining solution (microwave) hastens destaining considerably.

3. Store destained gels in sealed plastic bags or soak gels in 2% glycerol overnight, then sandwich between two cellophane sheets (BioRad #165-0922 or RPI #1080) without any bubbles on a open Plexiglass frame (RPI #1071) at room temperature.

Protein Silver Stain

Silver stains may be 100 times more sensitive than Coomassie blue, but require more attention and reagent preparation. The chemical basis for silver staining parallels photoreduced silver images in photography, but the precise interaction between protein and silver remains unknown. Apparently, the proteins in the gel act as reducing agents to catalyze the reduction of silver halide in the staining solution to metallic silver.

The staining procedure given here (adapted from Morrissey, 1981) is a neutral silver staining method; it is simple to use, sensitive to 10 ng of protein, and does not require precise volumes or times. An alternative silver stain that is slightly faster but not as sensitive is described by Bloom *et al.* (1987). Commercial silver staining kits are also available and offer maximum sensitivity (Pierce, Sigma, BioRad).

Reagents

Store all reagents at room temperature, except as noted.

Fix

    50% methanol
    10% acetic acid
    40% H_2O

Dithiothreitol (DTT Stock)

    5 mg/ml stock solution in water
    Store 25-μl samples frozen at −20°C.

Developer

    Mix the two reagents immediately before use.
    50 μl 37% formaldehyde
    100 ml 3% Na_2CO_3

Silver Nitrate Stock

10% silver nitrate in water
Store in an amber bottle.

Stop Solution

2.3 M citric acid

Procedure

1. Fix gel in fix solution for 15 min in a plastic or glass dish.

2. Rinse gel briefly with deionized water.

3. Dilute 10 μl DTT stock into 100 ml H_2O. Pour onto gel; shake 15–30 min.

4. Pour out DTT. Do not rinse gel.

5. Add 0.1% silver nitrate to gel (1 ml stock in 100 ml H_2O). Shake 15–30 min.

6. Pour off silver nitrate; rinse in H_2O. Add 25 ml developer. Shake 10–20 sec and pour off. Add 75 ml developer. Shake until developed (5–10 min).

7. Add 5 ml citric acid to stop. After 5 min, wash several times with water.

8. If background staining is high, reduce with a quick 15–30 sec wash in 1% Farmers reducer (available at photo stores). Wash again with water.

9. Dry gel after soaking in 2% glycerol (see Coomassie stain procedure, Step 3).

Carbohydrate Fluorescence Staining

Carbohydrate staining (Estep and Miller, 1986) is not as easy as protein staining. Carbohydrate does not bind dyes strongly enough to be visualized in the microgram range available on PAGE gels. Thus, more elaborate procedures must be done to achieve effective carbohydrate staining. In this procedure, glycoproteins in PAGE gels are first oxidized with periodate to generate aldehyde groups on the carbohydrate portions of the proteins. The aldehydes then are reacted with dansylhydrazine to form stable hydrazone bonds. The fluorescent dansyl–glycoproteins are visualized under ultraviolet light. This procedure is more sensitive than the older nonfluorescent periodic acid–Schiff stain (Zacharius *et al.*, 1969).

Reagents

Periodic Acid

 0.5% periodic acid, freshly made in deionized water

Sodium Metabisulfite

 0.5% sodium metabisulfite
 5% acetic acid

Sodium Acetate, pH 5.6

 0.1 M acetic acid
 Adjust pH to 5.6 with NaOH.

Dansyl Hydrazine

 0.1 gm dansyl hydrazine dissolved in 33 ml absolute ethanol
 67 ml 0.1 M acetate, pH 5.6
 Make this reagent immediately before use.

Sodium Borohydride

 0.2 gm NaBH4
 100 ml 0.1 M acetate, pH 5.6
 Make this reagent immediately before use.

Procedure

All steps are done at room temperature, for the time indicated.

1. Immerse gel in fresh 0.5% periodic acid (2 hr).

2. Rinse lightly with water (0.5 min).

3. Immerse gel in sodium metabisulfite (30 min).

4. Rinse three times with water (2 min).

5. Immerse gel in 100 ml dansyl hydrazine solution (2 hr).

6. Rinse with 0.1 M acetate, pH 5.6 (0.5 min).

7. Immerse in 100 ml 0.2% $NaBH_4$ (30 min).

8. Rinse twice with 1.0 M acetate, pH 5.6 (1 hr).

9. Visualize by illuminating with UV light.

Carbohydrate Enzyme Staining

This method (Clegg, 1982) is more sensitive than the fluorescent procedure, but more complicated because the proteins are electrotransferred to nitrocellulose membrane first. Next, concanavalin A is added, which binds to the glycoproteins. Finally, horseradish peroxidase is added, which binds to the concanavalin A because it, too, is a glycoprotein. The presence of peroxidase, which is bound to the glycoprotein, is detected with an insoluble chromogenic substrate. An alternate procedure based on binding peroxidase to polyhydrazide-modified glycoproteins claims to be more sensitive but requires synthesis of the polyhydrazide (Heimgartner *et. al.*, 1989).

Reagents

2% bovine serum albumin in water

TBS-Triton Buffer
0.01 M Tris, pH 7.4
0.15 M NaCl
10 μM $CaCl_2$
10 μM $MgCl_2$
0.1% Triton X-100
Ca and Mg are necessary for concanavalin A (Con-A) binding, but most Con-A preparations have bound cations and are active without added metals.

Concanavalin A

(Con-A; 15–25 ml required)

10 µg/ml concanavalin A in TBS-Triton buffer

Horseradish Peroxidase

50 µg/ml horseradish peroxidase in TBS-Triton buffer

(HRP, 15–25 ml required per membrane)

Chloronaphthol Developer

See Western Blot Reagents, Appendix D, p. 161.

Procedure

All steps are done at room temperature.

1. Transfer the proteins from the PAGE gel to nitrocellulose membrane. After the transfer, block with 2% bovine serum albumin for 1 hr.

2. Incubate the membrane for 1 hr with 15–25 ml Con-A.

3. Wash four times with TBS-Triton.

4. Incubate membrane for 1 hr with 15–25 ml HRP.

5. Wash four times with TBS-Triton and develop with chloronaphthol.

REFERENCES

Bloom, H., Beier, H., and Gross, H. S. (1987). Improved silver staining of plant proteins, RNA, and DNA in polyacrylamide gels. *Electrophoresis* **8**, 93–99.

Clegg, J. C. S. (1982). Glycoprotein detection in nitrocellulose transfers of electrophoretically separated protein mixtures using concanavalin A and peroxidase: Application to arenavirus and flavivirus proteins. *Anal. Biochem.* **127**, 389–394.

Daban, J.-R., Bartolome, S., and Samso, M. (1991). Use of the hydrophobic probe nile red for the fluorescent staining of protein bands in sodium dodecyl sulfate polyacrylamide gels. *Anal. Biochem.* **199**, 169–174.

Estep, T. N., and Miller, T. J. (1986). Optimization of erythrocyte membrane glycoprotein fluorescent labeling with dansylhydrazine after polyacrylamide gel electrophoresis. *Anal. Biochem.* **157**, 100–105.

Giulian, G. G., Moss, R. L., and Greaser, M. (1983). Improved methodology for analysis and quantitation of proteins on one-dimensional silver-stained slab gels. *Anal. Biochem.* **129**, 277–287.

Heimgartner, U., Kozulic, B., and Mosbach, K. (1989). Polyacrylic polyhydrazides as reagents for detection of glycoprotein. *Anal. Biochem.* **181**, 182–189.

Laemmli, U. K. (1970). Cleavage of structural proteins during the assembly of the head of bacteriophage T4. *Nature (London)* **227**, 680–685.

LeBlanc, G. A., and Cochrane, B. J. (1987). A rapid method for staining proteins in acrylamide gels. *Anal. Biochem.* **161**, 172–175.

Lee, C., Levin, A., and Branton, D. (1987). Copper staining: A five-minute protein stain for sodium dodecyl sulfate–polyacrylamide gels. *Anal. Biochem.* **166**, 308–312.

Merril, C. R., Goldman, D., and Van Keuren, M. L. (1984). Gel protein stains: Silver stain. *Meth. Enzymol.* **104**, 441–447.

Morrissey, J. H. (1981). Silver stain for proteins in polyacrylamide gels: A modified procedure with enhanced uniform sensitivity. *Anal. Biochem.* **117**, 307–310.

Zacharius, R. M., Zell, T. E., Morrison, J. H., and Woodlock, J. J. (1969). Glycoprotein staining following electrophoresis on acrylamide gels. *Anal. Biochem.* **30**, 148–152.

Western Blotting Reagents and Staining Procedures

ELECTROTRANSFER OF PROTEINS FROM PAGE GEL TO MEMBRANE

Materials

Transfer Buffer

☐ (25 mM Tris, 192 mM glycine, pH 8.3)

☐ 12.0 gm Tris base

☐ 57.6 gm glycine

☐ 800 ml methanol

☐ Bring volume up to 4 liters with water. Adjust pH to 8.1–8.3. Store at 4°C.

☐ Reuse 3–4 times. (From Towbin *et. al.*, 1979.)

Transfer Membrane

☐ cellulose nitrate membrane (Schleicher & Schuell, Optibind # 62940)
This membrane is supported with fibers and is very tear resistant.

☐ filter papers

☐ parafilm

Equipment

☐ blotting apparatus

☐ scotchbrite pads

☐ power supply

☐ tray

☐ weight

☐ glass plates

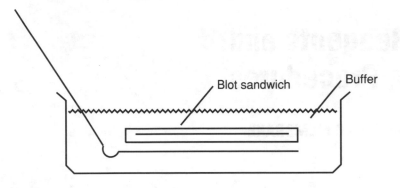

FIGURE 1

Forming the sandwich submerged in buffer.

Procedure

After PAGE, place the gel on a prewetted membrane totally submerged in transfer buffer held in a deep tray (Figure 1). Layer the gel, membrane, filter paper, and pads to form a sandwich, according to Figure 2. Take care to prewet all the components of the sandwich thoroughly and to eliminate all trapped air bubbles, which will cause white spots on the final blot because of incomplete transfer of protein. Once the sandwich has been assembled and is held together firmly, remove it

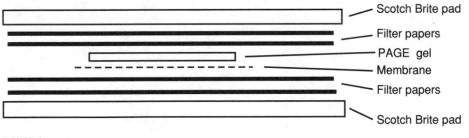

FIGURE 2

PAGE–membrane sandwich.

from the tray and immediately place it vertically in the transfer tank. Be sure the membrane side of the sandwich is facing the anode (+ pole) to insure the migration of proteins from the gel to the membrane.

Effective transfer will require 12–18 hr at 30 V or 1–2 hr at 70 V, assuming a 10-cm distance between electrodes. Stir the buffer during electrophoresis, if possible, to keep the concentration of migrating ions constant throughout the tank. When finished, remove the sandwich from the tank, peel it apart, and carefully lift the membrane and gel onto a piece of parafilm. Be sure to mark the corners of the gel before removing the gel from the membrane, and to identify any lanes directly on the membrane with a ball point pen.

CHLORONAPHTHOL STAIN FOR PEROXIDASE

Materials
□ 100 ml 0.05 M sodium or potassium phosphate, pH 6.5–6.8

□ 3% hydrogen peroxide (store in refrigerator)

□ ice cold methanol (store in −20°C freezer)

□ 4-chloro-1-naphthol (store dessicated in the dark in refrigerator)

Procedure
1. Place membrane face up in a shallow plastic dish.

2. Add 0.6 ml 3% hydrogen peroxide to 100 ml 0.05 M phosphate, pH 6.5–6.8.

3. Dissolve 60 mg 4-chloro-1-naphthol in 20 ml ice cold methanol. Immediately add to the phosphate–peroxide mixture, gently swirl, and pour onto the membrane.

4. Incubate at room temperature for 10–60 min with occasional gentle agitation. Watch for bands to appear! When the bands are dark enough, discard solution in carcinogenic waste.

5. Wash membrane three times with water.

6. Dry the membrane between filter paper under a glass plate with a weight on top. Store protected from light, otherwise the bands will fade. Photograph the membrane to obtain a permanent record.

AMIDOBLACK FOR PROTEIN STAINING ON NITROCELLULOSE MEMBRANE

Materials

□ 1 gm amidoblack (0.1%)

□ 450 ml methanol (45%)

□ 100 ml acetic acid (10%)

□ 450 ml distilled water

Mix well to dissolve and filter before use. Store in a dark bottle.

Procedure

1. Stain 3–5 min in shallow plastic dish.

2. Destain with repeated water washings until the background is white.

3. Dry between filter paper as in procedure 6, above. Store in the dark. Photograph membrane for a permanent record.

REFERENCE

Towbin, H., Staehelin, T., and Gordon, J. (1979). Electrophoretic transfer of proteins from polyacrylamide gels to nitrocelluose sheets: Procedure and some applications. *Proc. Natl. Acad. Sci. U.S.A.* **76**, 4350–4354.

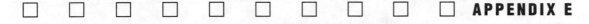
Suppliers of Equipment and Chemical Reagents

Directories of Suppliers

Linscott's Directory of Immunological and Biological Reagents
40 Glen Drive
Mill Valley, California 94941
415-383-2666

a reference source for many reagents, providing a listing of reagents and the companies that supply them (addresses included)

Suppliers of Antibodies, Custom Antibody Services, and Immunological Reagents

Accurate Chemical and Scientific Corp.
300 Shames Drive
Westbury, New York 11590
800-645-6264 (East); 800-255-9378 (West)
516-333-2221 (East); 619-235-9400 (West)

antibodies, complement, cell typing antisera

Biodesign International
432 Beachweed Avenue
Kennebunkport, Maine 04046
207-967-4173

antibodies, custom antibodies

Cappel Research Products
Organon Teknika Corp.
100 Akzo Avenue
Durham, North Carolina 27704
800-523-7620; 919-620-2107

antibodies, labeled antibodies, immunological reagents

Chemicon International, Inc.
27515 Enterprise Circle West
Temecula, California 92390
714-676-9209

antibodies, custom antibodies

Jackson Immunoresearch Labs, Inc.
P.O. Box 9
West Grove, Pennsylvania 19390
800-367-5296, 215-869-4024

antibodies, labeled antibodies,
immunological reagents, pure
immunoglobulins

Pel-Freez Biologicals
P.O. Box 68
205 N. Arkansas St.
Rogers, Arkansas 72757
800-643-3426, 501-636-4361

custom antibody service, blood,
complement, serum, tissues, organs,
pure immunoglobulins

Sigma Chemical Company
P.O. Box 14508
St. Louis, Missouri 63178
800-325-8070

general organic biochemicals, immunological
reagents, radioisotopes, cell culture

Vector Laboratories, Inc.
30 Ingold Road
Burlingame, California 94010
415-697-3600

labeled immunological reagents, some
antibodies

Zymed Laboratories Inc.
52 S. Linden Avenue # 1
South San Francisco, California 94080
800-874-4494 (outside California), 415-871-4494

immunological reagents, some antibodies

Suppliers of Blood, Blood Products, Animals, and Tissues

Colorado Serum Company
4950 York Street
P.O. Box 16428
Denver, Colorado 80216
303-295-7527

blood, complement, serum

Pel-Freez Biologicals
P.O. Box 68
205 N. Arkansas St.
Rogers, Arkansas 72757
800-643-3426, 501-636-4361

blood, complement, serum, tissues,
organs, pure immunoglobulins, custom
antibody service

Rockland, Inc.
  Box 316
  Gilbertsville, Pennsylvania 19525
  215-369-1008

blood, antibodies, complement, serum,
tissues, pure immunoglobulins, animals

Suppliers of Instrumentation

Beckman Instruments, Inc.
  Diagnostic Systems Group
  200 S. Kraemer Blvd.
  Brea, California 92621-6209
  714-993-5321

immunoelectrophoresis apparatus,
microfuges

BioRad Laboratories
  3300 Regatta Blvd.
  Richmond, California 94804
  800-227-5589; 800-2273259 (in California)
  85A Marcus Dr.
  Melville, New York 11747
  800-645-3227; 800-632-3060 (in New York)

electrophoresis, transfer apparatus,
chromatography, multichannel
micropipets

E-C Apparatus
  3831 Tyrone Blvd. North
  Saint Petersburg, Florida 33709
  800-327-2643, 813-344-1644

immunoelectrophoresis

Flow Laboratories Inc.
  7655 Old Springhouse Road
  McLean, Virginia 22102
  800-368-3569; 703-893-5925

microtiter ELISA plate reader,
multichannel micropipets

Gelman Sciences
  600 S. Wagner Road
  Ann Arbor, Michigan 48106
  800-521-1520; 313-665-0651

cellulose acetate electrophoresis

Helena Laboratories
  1530 Lindbergh Drive
  P.O. Box 752
  Beumont, Texas 77704-0752
  800-231-5663; 409-842-3714

immunoelectrophoresis, cellulose acetate
electrophoresis

Hoefer Scientific Instruments   electrophoresis, transfer apparatus
654 Minnesota Street, Box 77387
San Francisco, California 94107
800-227-4750; 415-282-2307

Idea Scientific Company   electrophoresis, transfer apparatus
P.O. Box 13210
Minneapolis, Minnesota 55414
612-331-4612

RPI, Research Products International   PAGE gel drying frames, miscellaneous
410 N. Business Center Drive   plasticware
Mt. Prospect, Illinois 60056
800-323-9814

Suppliers of Chemicals and Miscellaneous Reagents

Amersham Corporation   isotopes, radiolabeled antibodies and
2636 South Clarbrook Drive   immunological reagents, radiographic
Arlington Heights, Illinois 60005   cassettes and films
800-323-9750; 312-354-7100

Pierce Chemical Company   immunological reagents, protein
P.O. Box 117   modification reagents
Rockford, Illinois 61105
800-874-3723

ICN Biomedicals, Inc.   general organic biochemicals, immunological
3300 Hyland Avenue   reagents, radioisotopes, cell culture
Costa Mesa, California 92626
800-854-0530

Sigma Chemical Company   general biochemicals, immunological
P.O. Box 14508   reagents, radioisotopes, cell culture
St. Louis, Missouri 63178
800-325-8070

Saturated Ammonium Sulfate Table

Milligrams of Solid Ammonium Sulfate to Add to 1 ml Solution to Achieve Desired Percentage Saturation at 0°C

Initial percentage of ammonium sulfate	Final percentage of ammonium sulfate in solution at 0°C																
	20	25	30	35	40	45	50	55	60	65	70	75	80	85	90	95	100
0	106	134	164	194	226	258	291	326	361	398	436	476	516	559	603	630	697
5	79	108	137	166	197	229	262	296	331	368	405	444	484	526	570	615	662
10	53	81	109	139	169	200	233	266	301	337	374	412	452	493	536	581	627
15	26	54	82	111	141	172	204	237	271	316	343	381	420	460	503	547	592
20	0	27	55	83	113	143	175	207	241	276	312	349	387	427	469	512	557
25		0	27	56	84	115	146	179	211	245	280	317	365	395	436	488	522
30			0	28	56	86	117	148	181	214	249	285	323	362	402	445	488
35				0	28	57	87	118	151	184	218	254	291	329	369	410	453
40					0	29	58	89	120	153	182	212	258	296	335	376	418
45						0	29	59	90	123	156	190	226	263	302	342	383
50							0	30	60	92	125	159	194	230	268	308	348
55								0	30	61	93	127	161	197	235	273	313
60									0	31	62	95	129	164	201	239	279
65										0	31	63	97	132	168	205	244
70											0	32	65	99	134	171	209
75												0	32	66	101	137	174
80													0	33	67	103	139
85														0	34	68	105
90															0	34	70
95																0	35
100																	0

Radioiodination of Proteins

Advantages of Radioiodination

Radioactive iodine is probably the most common *in vitro* radiolabel for proteins. Both ^{125}I and ^{131}I are γ emitters and are detected easily by NaI crystal scintillation counters or by radiographic techniques. The relatively short half-life (60 days for ^{125}I and 8 days for ^{131}I) allows proteins to be labeled to high specific activities, and the labeling procedures are simple and reproducible. ^{125}I usually is chosen for research laboratory iodination because it has a longer half-life, is counted at a higher efficiency, and is available at a higher radionuclide purity. Therapeutic and clinical applications often use the higher specific activities and shorter half-life offered by ^{131}I. If iodination is not compatible with a particular protein or technique, radiolabeling with ^3H or ^{14}C is possible by reductive methylation (Dattavio-Martin and Joanne, 1978; Jentoft and Dearborn, 1980) However, the lower specific activities and long half-lifes of these isotopes limits their usefulness and necessitates counting with liquid scintillation fluors, creating both additional steps and long-lived radioactive organic waste.

Chemistry of Iodination

Iodine is introduced into a protein by one of two methods: direct iodination using oxidizing agents or indirectly using an intermediate iodinated molecule (for review, see Parker, 1990). The direct methods oxidize $Na^{125}I$ to form a cationic iodointermediate, I^+, probably in the form of I_2 or ICl, which then substitutes *ortho* to the hydroxyl group on tyrosine and, to a lesser extent, on histidine and tryptophan. Oxidation is accomplished by chemical treatment (chloramine-T; Hunter and Greenwood, 1962) or by enzymatic means (lactoperoxidase; Marchalonis, 1969; David and Reisfeld, 1974). Compared with the lactoperoxidase procedure, the chloramine-T procedure may produce di-iodotyrosine and may cause more oxidative protein damage, but often labels to a higher specific activity. If mono-iodotyrosine labels are required, or if the protein is sensitive to oxidative damage, lactoperoxidase may be preferred. However, not all proteins label well using the enzyme procedure, since surface tyrosines on the protein may not be labeled effectively by the enzyme.

The second method of iodination uses an intermediate iodinated molecule that attaches to the protein, obviating the need to expose the protein to oxidation. The most common intermediate label is the Bolton–Hunter reagent (Bolton and Hunter, 1973), which attaches to primary amino groups on the protein. The reagent, 3-(*p*-hydroxyphenyl)-propionic acid-*N*-hydroxysuccinimide, is first iodinated on the hydroxyphenyl group with chloramine-T, then attached to free amino groups on the protein through the succinimidyl ester. Para-hydroxyphenylacetaldehyde is an alternative intermediate molecule that requires mild reduction with sodium cyanoborohydride to form a covalent bond with primary amino groups (Panuska and Parker, 1987). These intermediates do not affect tyrosines on proteins, but do substitute positive amino groups with potentially negative phenolic hydroxyl groups. Indirect labeling often results in lower specific activities than direct iodination, but may be necessary for proteins with few or critical tyrosines.

Chloramine-T Iodination Procedure

The procedure presented here uses chloramine-T and $Na^{125}I$ to label proteins. During the procedure, any excess volatile ^{125}I is reacted with excess tyrosine, and ^{125}I-labeled protein is separated from this and other low molecular weight compounds by gel filtration. No reducing agent such as sodium metabisulfite is used to stop the oxidation, because it is known to damage proteins. For convenience, solid-state reagents that are chloramine-T derivatives (Iodo-Gen and Iodo-Beads, Pierce) or solid-phase lactoperoxidase (Enzymobead, BioRad) offer the advantage of being ready to use, but still require separation of free from bound iodine.

Materials

□ chloramine-T (Sigma), 2 mg/ml in 0.30 M phosphate, pH 7.3
  Make immediately before use.

□ tyrosine, 0.3 mg/ml in 0.30 M phosphate, pH 7.3
  This is a saturated solution of tyrosine.

□ protein, 1–5 mg/ml in dilute phosphate buffer, pH 6–8

□ 0.5–1.0 mCi ^{125}I, carrier free (as Na^{125}I in NaOH; Amersham #IMS.30)

□ PBS (Appendix B)

□ 5% bovine serum albumin

□ 5-ml column of Sephadex G-25 in PBS, precoated with 1 ml 5% bovine
  serum albumin and washed with 4 column volumes of PBS
    This column is conveniently made in a disposable 5-ml glass or plastic
  pipet.

□ lead bricks or lead shield set in a well-ventilated fume hood with absorbent
  towels

□ micropipets

□ radioactive waste disposal bags

□ radiation survey meter

Procedure

During the activation, volatile ^{125}I$_2$ is formed which must be removed effectively
by a well-ventilated fume hood. Gloves should be worn during all handling of isotopes, since iodine is absorbed effectively by the skin. All waste must be marked
clearly with type of isotope, approximate quantity, and date of use. Survey the area
after iodination to detect any spilled isotope. A pristine work place should be the
goal after the iodination, and careful attention must be paid to organizing and
having available all necessary equipment and reagents *before* the iodination. Any
person who performs radioiodinations regularly should have twice-yearly thyroid
scans to see if significant ^{125}I has accumulated.

1. Add, in order, to a 10×75-mm *glass* tube 0.010 ml chloramine-T, 0.010 ml 0.3 M phosphate, pH 7.3, 0.005–0.010 ml carrier-free ^{125}I, and 0.010 ml protein.

2. Incubate at room temperature for 2 min.

3. Add 0.025 ml tyrosine. Incubate at room temperature for 2 min.

4. Add 0.050 ml 5% BSA (may be omitted if iodinated protein must not be contaminated with BSA) and 0.200 ml PBS.

5. Apply mixture to a 5-ml Sephadex G-25 column that has been drained to form a "dry" bed top. After all mixture has entered the column, wash the sides of the column with 0.200 ml PBS, followed by 1.0 ml PBS. Discard all eluate up to this point.

6. Elute the labeled protein by adding an additional 1.0 ml PBS and collecting the resulting 1.0 ml eluate. The ^{125}I-labeled protein should be eluted in this fraction, whereas unbound ^{125}I should still be retained on the column. If desired, additional 0.5-ml fractions may be collected to verify recovery of the labeled protein.

7. Take a small amount of the labeled protein solution (5–10 μl) and count in a NaI scintillation counter to determine the specific activity.

REFERENCES

Bolton, A. E., and Hunter, W. M. (1973). The labelling of proteins to high specific radioactivities by conjugation to a ^{125}I-containing acylating agent. *Biochem. J.* **133**, 529–539.

Dattavio-Martin, D., and Joanne, R. M. (1978). Radiolabeling of proteins by reductive methylation with ^{14}C-formaldehyde and sodium borohydride. *Anal. Biochem.* **87**, 562–565.

David, G. S., and Reisfeld, R. A. (1974). Protein iodination with solid state lactoperoxidase. *Biochemistry* **13**, 1014–1021.

Hunter, W. M., and Greenwood, F. C. (1962). Preparation of iodine-131 labelled human growth hormone of high specific activity. *Nature (London)* **194**, 495–496.

Jentoft, J., and Dearborn, D. G. (1980). Protein labeling by reductive methylation with sodium cyanoborohydride and effect of cyanide and metal ions on the reaction. *Anal. Biochem.* **106** 186–190.

Marchalonis, J. J. (1969). An enzymic method for the trace iodination of immunoglobulins and other proteins. *Biochem. J.* **113**, 299–305.

Panuska, J. R., and Parker, C. W. (1987). Radioiodination of proteins by reductive alkylation. *Anal. Biochem.* **160**, 192–201.

Parker, C. W. (1990). Radiolabeling of proteins. *Meth. Enzymol.* **182**, 721–737.

Immunization Procedure

Use of Adjuvants during Immunization

The response of an animal to an antigen depends on an involved leukocyte–antigen interaction. The antigen is recognized by specialized B and T lymphocytes and the sustained presence of the antibody-producing B-cells depends strongly on subsequent macrophage (or antigen-presenting cell) interaction with lymphocytes over a period of time. Thus, good immunization protocols require both the sustained localization of antigen, and the recruitment of appropriate leukocytes to the antigen. To achieve this goal, substances termed *adjuvants* are used during the immunization procedure. These substances localize at the point of injection, providing a low but consistent presence of antigen in the animal that stimulates the production of antibody. The most popular adjuvant for protein immunization is probably Freund's adjuvant. This mineral oil-based adjuvant comes in two versions, with (complete) or without (incomplete) killed *Mycobacterium tuberculosis* bacteria. The adjuvant is emulsified with the aqueous antigen and injected subcutaneously or intramuscularly to deposit the antigen. The oils in the emulsion are not metabolized and slowly leak the antigen to the immune system of the animal. Further, the presence of *M. tuberculosis* cells stimulates the cells of the immune system, enhancing the specific response to the antigen. The disadvantage of Freund's adjuvant is the possible formation of granulomas at the site of injection, which may blister and become infected, causing discomfort to the animal. However, if used properly, little or no toxic side effects result from Freund's. Injecting only small, 25–100 μl doses of complete Freund's at multiple sites results in sustained high titers without the need for frequent boosting. If necessary, subsequent boosts are done with incomplete Freund's, which produces less toxicity. A new commercial adjuvant, TiterMax, (CytRx Corporation, Technology Park, Atlanta, Georgia) is claimed to provide a prolonged high titer response with minimal toxic effects in rodents. At this time little is known about its effectiveness in larger animals.

Freund's adjuvant water-in-oil emulsions are prepared most efficiently by connecting two syringes with a two-way luer fitting. (A 3-way stopcock luer fitting works well.) To prepare 2 ml emulsion, half fill a 2-ml glass syringe with 1 ml Freund's adjuvant, attach to one of the luer fittings, and connect the other 2-ml syringe filled with 1 ml antigen to the other half of the luer fitting. The *aqueous* solution then is pushed quickly into the *oil*, and the mixture is pushed back and forth for 2–3 min. This produces a water-in-oil emulsion that is most stable. A stable emulsion must be obtained before injecting and may be tested by dripping one drop into a beaker of clean water. The first drop will spread across the surface, but the second drop should remain predominantly as a single spot without significant spreading. Plastic syringes do not work in the emulsification process since the plungers seize in the barrels after repeated movement. If a stable emulsion cannot be obtained, then perhaps the antigen buffer is too high in salt (>1 M) or a detergent is present. It is preferable to have the antigen in 0.15 M NaCl with either phosphate or Tris buffering to a pH of 6–8. A second method to prepare an emulsion is to vortex vigorously a 1:1 mixture of adjuvant and aqueous antigen. It is more difficult to obtain a stable emulsion by this method, but it is useful if less than one millimeter of immunogen is being prepared.

Immunization Protocol

The amount of protein antigen needed for the production of 1 liter of antiserum from a sheep or goat is 0.5–5 mg. Rabbits may require more antigen because of the longer immunization period required to obtain sufficient antiserum. The protocol described here has worked well with a number of protein antigens of different molecular weights and species of origin. However, if the antigen is in low supply, considerably smaller amounts of antigen will provide a good response also. However, antibody production may not be as consistently high, and may require more frequent boosts. Subcutaneous injections (SC) are made by pinching the skin and pulling up about 1 cm, and then injecting the antigen between the fold of skin at the base of the pinch. The antigen should form a slight pool immediately underneath the skin, not in the body wall. Subcutaneous injections are done at a variety of locations on the animal, including above the shoulders, along the flank, and along the back. Intramuscular injections (IM) deposit the antigen in the flesh of the muscle, about 1 cm deep. Injection sites include the shoulder and thigh muscles. Use 21–23 gauge needles for all injections, and be sure to change needles between animals. Injections should follow the schedule given in Table 1.

Test bleeds are obtained from the jugular vein on the neck of the goat or sheep. If you are unfamiliar with bleeding, enlist the services of an animal care technician or a veterinarian. See the experimental sections for obtaining serum from blood (Experiment 1) and testing the antiserum by Ouchterlony double diffusion (Experiment 4).

Injection Schedule

Day	Type of Injection and Adjuvant
0	SC, 10–20 sites, each with 0.05 ml of 1.0 mg/ml antigen in complete Freund's
21	Test bleed: check for antibody by agarose double diffusion
28	Bleed every 5–7 days for antibody collection if response is adequate
	Continue to boost as needed (IM, 8–10 sites, each with 0.1 ml of 1.0 mg/ml antigen in incomplete Freund's) to maintain high titer antiserum. Bleed 5–7 days after boost to determine response.

REFERENCE

Herbert, W. J., and Kristensen, F. (1986). Laboratory animal techniques for immunology. *In* Handbook of Experimental Immunology, 4th edition (D. M. Wier, ed.) Vol 4, 133.1–133.36. Blackwell, Oxford.

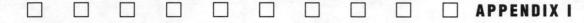

Detergent Solubilization of Proteins

Detergents are molecules with hydrophobic and hydrophilic portions useful to purify and study membrane proteins. The detergents act both to disrupt the lipid bilayer membrane and to solubilize the released proteins. During solubilization, the detergent binds to hydrophobic areas on proteins that were formerly occupied by membrane lipids. Once solubilized, the protein–detergent complex forms a *micelle*, a colloidal-sized structure composed of many detergent molecules with their hydrophobic portions on the inside and hydrophilic portions on the outside. Usually several proteins are inserted in each micelle. For membrane protein isolation, it is best to keep the detergent:lipid ratio above 10–20, insuring that the isolated protein is free of lipids. A schematic of the events that occur during membrane disruption is given in Figure 1.

Several characteristics of detergents should be considered when solubilizing proteins. The critical micelle concentration (CMC) is the concentration at which

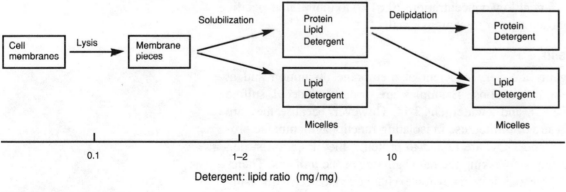

FIGURE 1

Membrane disruption. Adapted from Helenius *et al.* (1979).

free detergent monomers form micelles. In general, a high CMC is desired if excess detergent is to be removed by dialysis. (A low CMC means micelles easily form that are difficult to dialyze.) The micelles are further defined both by their size and by the number of monomers per micelle, the *aggregation number*. A small aggregation number is preferred if structural or molecular weight studies are to be done; the protein characteristics are altered least with a minimum number of detergent molecules bound. Finally, if detergent-solubilized proteins are purified further by chromatographic or electrophoretic techniques, nondenaturing detergents must be used to preserve enzymatic activity and native protein structure. A researcher must be aware of possible effects of the detergent on the charge properties of the isolated proteins, the formation of artificial protein–detergent aggregates, and the dissociation of detergents from isolated proteins. A few of the common detergents are discussed in the following sections. For detergent parameters, see Table 1.

Nonionic Polyoxyethylene Ether Detergents

Nonionic polyoxethylene ether detergents are electrically neutral. Examples are Triton X-100, Lubrol PX, and Nonidet-40. Although they are mild enough to isolate functional membrane proteins, their low CMC and high affinities for proteins make them difficult to separate from proteins. These detergents also commonly are incorporated into buffers at low concentrations (0.01%) to inhibit nonspecific binding of proteins to one another or to container walls.

Anionic *N*-Alkyl Detergents

Anionic *N*-alkyl detergents are very efficient at membrane disruption and at breaking protein–protein interactions. Examples are sodium dodecyl sulfate (SDS), deoxycholate (DOC), and Zwittergent 3-14. However, because they are strongly denaturing, they are of limited use in isolating functional membrane proteins. Further, when SDS and DOC are bound to proteins, they impart a strong negative charge to the proteins, masking the native charge of the proteins. Therefore, fractionation of SDS-treated proteins by ion exchange or isoelectric focusing is difficult or impossible.

TABLE 1

Detergents Useful for Sample Solubilization

Structural formula	Chemical or trade name	CMC	Micellar weight	Aggregation number
Anionic detergents				
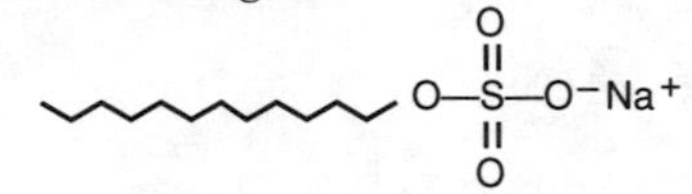	Sodium dodecyl sulfate (SDS)	2–10 mM	18,000 to 36,000	60–100
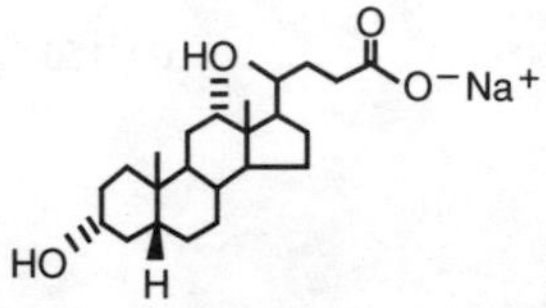	Sodium deoxycholate (DOC)	2 to 6 mM	1,700 to 4,200	4 to 10
Cationic detergent				
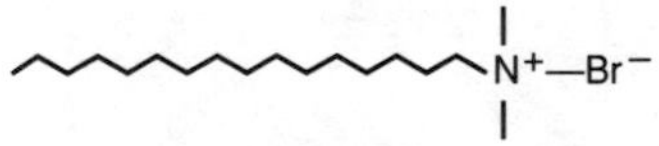	Cetyltrimethylammonium bromide	—	62,000	170
Zwitterionic detergent				
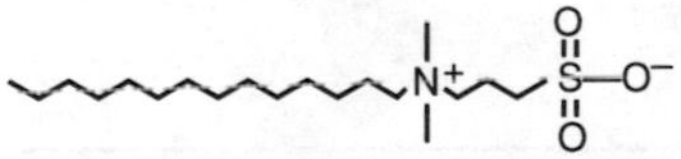	Zwittergent 3-14	0.1–0.4 mM	~ 30,000	50–80
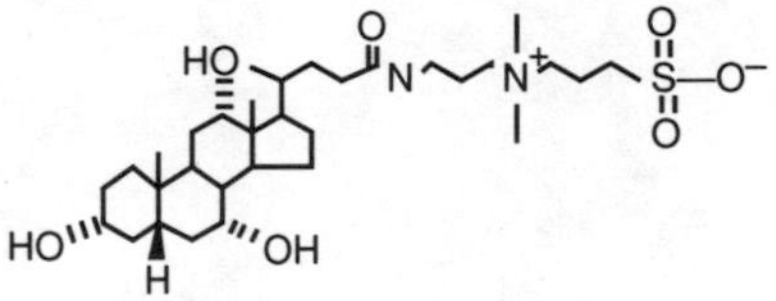	CHAPS	3–10 mM	—	10
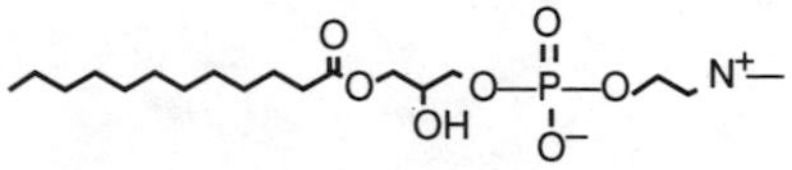	Lysophosphatidylcholine	0.9 mM	92,000	180

(continues)

TABLE 1   (*continued*)

Structural formula	Chemical or trade name	CMC	Micellar weight	Aggregation number
Nonionic Detergents				
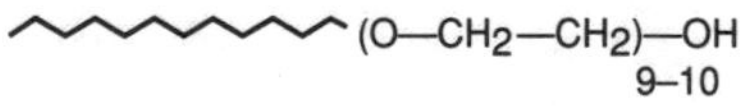 (O—CH₂—CH₂)—OH 9–10	Lubrol PX	0.10 mM	64,000	110
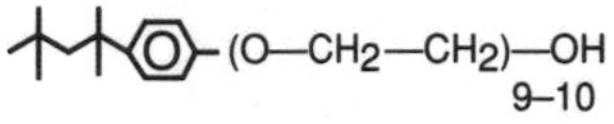 (O—CH₂—CH₂)—OH 9–10	Triton X-100 (NP-40)	0.29–0.9 mM	90,000	100–150
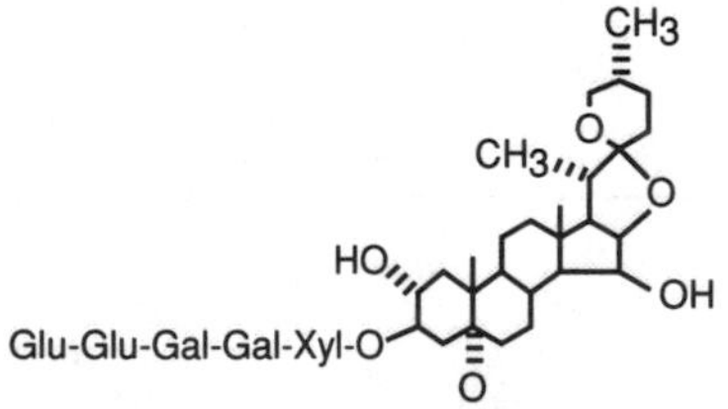 Glu-Glu-Gal-Gal-Xyl-O	Digitonin	—	70,000	60
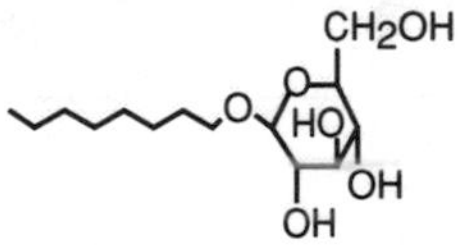	Octyl glucose (octyl-β–D-glucopyranoside)	25 mM	—	80

182

CHAPS and Octyl Glucose

These detergents are perhaps the best known to date for effectively isolating functional membrane proteins. Since they possess no net charge between pH 2 and 12, they do not affect the native charge of the protein, allowing purifications based on protein charge. Finally, since the CMCs are high for these detergents (6–25 mM), they usually can be removed readily by dialysis.

REFERENCES

Furth, A., Bolton, H., Potter, J., and Priddle, J. D. (1984). Separating detergent from proteins. *Meth. Enzymol.* **104**, 318–328.

Helenius, A., McCaslin, D. R., Fries, E., and Tanford, C. (1979). Properties of detergents. *Meth. Enzymol.* **56**, 734–749.

Hjelmeland, L. M. (1990). Solubilization of native membrane proteins. *Meth. Enzymol.* **182**, 253–265.

Index

Page numbers with an *mn* indicate a marginal note, those with a *t* indicate a table.